The Comfort of Home™

for Alzheimer's Disease

A Guide for Caregivers

The *Comfort of Home*™ Caregiver book series is written for family and paraprofessional home caregivers who face the responsibilities of caring for aging friends, family, or clients. The disease-specific editions, often in collaboration with organizations supporting those conditions, address caregivers assisting people with those diseases.

Other Caregiver Resources from CareTrust Publications:

La comodidad del hogar™ *(Spanish Edition)*
The Comfort of Home™: *A Complete Guide for Caregivers*
The Comfort of Home™ *for Chronic Lung Disease*
The Comfort of Home™ *for Chronic Heart Failure*
The Comfort of Home™ *for Chronic Liver Disease*
The Comfort of Home™ *Multiple Sclerosis Edition*
The Comfort of Home™ *for Parkinson Disease*
The Comfort of Home™ *for Stroke*
The Comfort of Home™ *Caregiving Journal*
The Comfort of Home™ *Caregivers—Let's Take Care of You!* Meditation CD

Newsletters:

The Comfort of Home™ *Caregiver Assistance News*
The Comfort of Home™ *Grand-Parenting News*
The Comfort of Home™ *Caregivers—Let's Take Care of You!*

Visit *www.comfortofhome.com* for forthcoming editions and other caregiver resources.

The Comfort of Home™

for Alzheimer's Disease

A Guide for Caregivers

Maria M. Meyer

Mary S. Mittelman, DrPH

Cynthia Epstein, LCSW

and

Paula Derr, RN, BSN, CEN, CCRN

CareTrust Publications LLC
"Caring for you...caring for others."
Portland, Oregon

Published by: CareTrust Publications LLC
P.O. Box 10283
Portland, Oregon 97296-0283
(800) 565-1533
Fax (503) 221-7019

Publisher's Cataloging-in-Publication
(Provided by Quality Books, Inc.)

Meyer, Maria M., 1948-
   The comfort of home for Alzheimer's disease : a guide
for caregivers / Maria M. Meyer, Mary S. Mittelman,
Cynthia Epstein and Paula Derr.
      p. cm.
   Includes index.
   ISBN-13: 978-0-9787903-0-1
   ISBN-10: 0-9787903-0-8

   1. Home care services—Handbooks, manuals, etc.
2. Caregivers—Handbooks, manuals, etc. 3. Alzheimer's
disease. I. Mittelman, Mary S. II. Epstein, Cynthia.
III. Derr, Paula. IV. Title.

RA645.3.M493 2008   649.8
                                     QBI07-600342

Cover Art and Text Illustration: Stacey L. Tandberg
Interior Design: Frank Loose
Cover Design: David Kessler
Page Layout: International Graphic Services

Distributed to the Trade by Publishers Group West.
Printed in the United States of America.

08 09 10 11 12 / 10 9 8 7 6 5 4 3 2 1

About the Authors

Maria M. Meyer has been a long-time advocate of social causes, beginning with her work as co-founder of the Society for Abused Children of the Children's Home Society of Florida and founding executive director of the Children's Foundation of Greater Miami. When her father-in-law suffered a stroke in 1993, Maria became aware of the need for better information about how to care for an aging parent, a responsibility shared by millions of Americans. That experience led Maria to found CareTrust Publications and to co-author the award-winning guide, *The Comfort of Home™: An Illustrated Step-by-Step Guide for Caregivers*—now in its third edition. This book earned the Benjamin Franklin Award in the health category. She is a keynote speaker and workshop leader on caregiver topics to health care professionals and community groups, as well as a Caregiver Community Action Network volunteer for the National Family Caregiver Association.

Mary S. Mittelman, DrPH, is an epidemiologist who has been evaluating psychosocial interventions for family members of people with Alzheimer's disease for the past two decades. She is Director of the Psychosocial Research and Support Program at the Silberstein Institute, Research Professor in the Department of Psychiatry at New York University School of Medicine, and leader of the Education and Psychosocial Cores of the NYU Alzheimer's Disease Center. She is Principal Investigator of the NYU-Spouse Caregiver Intervention study, funded by the NIH since 1987, as well as other studies of psychosocial interventions for people with cognitive impairment, dementia, and their family members. In the past few years, Dr. Mittelman has made a commitment to disseminate research findings to both health care providers and the community at large and to collaborate with researchers and community organizations to implement and test psychosocial interventions.

Cynthia Epstein, LCSW, a social worker and clinical investigator, is a graduate of the Hunter/Mt. Sinai Geriatric Education Center and the Brookdale Post Masters Program in Aging. For more than ten years she has counseled family caregivers and people with Alzheimer's disease who seek cognitive evaluations and participate in psychosocial interventions at the NYU Aging and Dementia Research Center. In addition to providing clinical supervision to social work students, many of whom are now Alzheimer's care providers themselves, she offers workshops for professional and family caregivers under the auspices of the New York City Alzheimer's Association. In her private psychotherapy practice she works with people coping with Alzheimer's-related issues as well as a range of other emotional concerns.

Paula Derr, RN, BSN, CEN, CCRN, has been employed by the Sisters of Providence Health System for over 30 years. She has broad experience in many different clinical settings and for many years served as clinical educator for three emergency departments in the Portland metropolitan area. She was a founder of inforMed, which publishes emergency medical services field guides for emergency medical technicians (EMTs), paramedics, firefighters, physicians, and nurses and has co-authored numerous health care articles. For Paula, home care is a family tradition of long standing. For many years, Paula cared for her mother and grandmother in her home while raising two daughters and maintaining her career in nursing and health care management. Her personal and professional experience adds depth to many chapters of this book. Paula is active in several prominent professional organizations and has held both local and national board positions. Paula is a native Oregonian and lives with her husband in Portland.

Our Mission

CareTrust Publications is committed to providing high-quality,
user-friendly information to those who face an illness or the
responsibilities of caring for friends, family, or clients.

Dedication

We dedicate this book to all the family caregivers and their relatives with
Alzheimer's disease who shared their experiences with us. Their strength
in facing and living with illness reveals the nobility and vulnerabilty that
constitute the essence of the human condition.

Dear Caregiver,

Caring for someone with Alzheimer's disease can be deeply satisfying as well as uniquely challenging. When they support each other in caring for someone who is ill, partners, family, and friends can be drawn more closely together. Yet, caregiving can also be physically and emotionally exhausting, especially for the person who is the primary caregiver.

The Comfort of Home™ *for Alzheimer's Disease: A Guide for Caregivers* is a basic, complete guide that will answer your questions about caregiving. Covering current best practices for home care, it offers practical tips for everyday problems as well as more complicated and stressful situations.

Even though Alzheimer's is a medical illness, its treatment is almost entirely based on caring and support. This book will tell you what you need to know so that you and the person with Alzheimer's disease can experience the coming years in the best way possible.

The *Guide* is divided into three parts:

Part One, Getting Ready, describes the stages of Alzheimer's disease and how the disease affects the person for whom you care. You will learn how to make the home safe and comfortable. There is information about getting the best home care and financial advice and making important decisions about the future, as well as how to maintain the physical and emotional health of the person with dementia.

Part Two, Day-by-Day Living with Alzheimer's Disease, tells you how to communicate effectively, develop a daily schedule, and understand the changing behaviors of the person with Alzheimer's disease while never losing sight of your own needs.

Part Three, Additional Resources, provides a glossary of common medical terms to help you understand the language that many health care professionals use to talk about Alzheimer's disease. It also includes a list of references for further reading and information about organizations and publications for caregivers.

Armed with knowledge, you will feel confident that you can provide good care. With this *Guide* in hand, you will understand what help is needed and learn where to find it or how to provide it yourself.

Warm regards,

Maria, Mary, Cynthia, and Paula

Acknowledgments

The information in this *Guide* is based on research and consultation with experts in the fields of nursing, medicine, and design. The authors thank the innumerable professionals and caregivers who have assisted in the development of this book.

This volume would not have been possible without the support of the Alzheimer's Association. They very generously allowed us access to their information, which details the most recent approaches to helping those living with Alzheimer's disease and their families.

We are grateful for the generous sharing of expertise by the NYU Alzheimer's Disease Center (supported by the NIA, grant number 5 P30 AG 008051). The NIMH (R01 MH 42216) and NIA (R01 AG14634) have been supportive in funding the long-running study of counseling and support of spouse caregivers that has provided the foundation for our work. We would also like to thank the Alzheimer's Association, the Langeloth Foundation, and Pfizer Inc. for the grant support that has enabled us to develop and test additional interventions for people with Alzheimer's disease and their family members. All the study participants merit a special "thank you." We hope the knowledge we have gained and offered in this book will inform, support, and bring comfort to its readers.

Special thanks go to the following people who shared their expertise in caring for those with dementia. They kindly offered materials and support:

Lisa P. Gwyther, MCW, LCSW
Education Director
Bryan Alzheimer's Disease Research
  Center
Duke University Medical Center

Daniel Kuhn, MSW
Director
Professional Training Institute
Alzheimer's Association—Greater Illinois
  Chapter

Teepa Snow, MS, OTR/L FAOTA
Eastern North Carolina Alzheimer's
  Association

Some sections of this volume are adapted from other editions in the *Comfort of Home*™ series. We extend our gratitude to those authors and organizations whose contributions have enhanced this book.

Beth Boyd-Roberts, PT
Physical Therapy–In-Patient Supervisor

Ray Jordan, CPA

James L. Meyer, AIA

Donald E. Nielsen, AIA

Northwest Parish Nurses Board of Directors

Annette Stixrud, RN, MS
Program Director
Northwest Parish Nurse Ministries

To Our Readers

We believe *The Comfort of Home™ for Alzheimer's Disease: A Guide for Caregivers* reflects currently accepted practice in the areas it covers. However, the authors and publisher assume no liability with respect to the accuracy, completeness, or application of information presented here.

The Comfort of Home™ for Alzheimer's Disease is not meant to replace medical care but to add to the medical advice and services you receive from health care professionals. You should seek professional medical advice from a health care provider. This book is only a guide; follow your common sense and good judgment.

Neither the authors nor the publisher are engaged in rendering legal, accounting, or other professional advice. Seek the services of a competent professional if legal, architectural, or other expert assistance is required. The *Guide* does not represent Americans with Disabilities Act compliance.

Every effort has been made at the time of publication to provide accurate names, addresses, and phone numbers in the resource sections at the ends of chapters. The resources listed are those that benefit readers nationally. For this reason we have not included many local groups that offer valuable assistance. Failure to include an organization does not mean that it does not provide a valuable service. On the other hand, inclusion does not imply an endorsement. The authors and publisher do not warrant or guarantee any of the products described in this book and did not perform any independent analysis of the products described.

Throughout the book, we use "he" and "she" interchangeably when referring to the caregiver and the person being cared for.

CONTENTS AT A GLANCE

Part Three   *Additional Resources*

Praise for *The Comfort of Home*™ Caregiver Guides

"This is an invaluable addition to bibliographies for the home caregiver. Hospital libraries will want to have a copy on hand for physicians, nurses, social workers, chaplains, and any staff dealing with MS patients and their caregivers. Highly recommended for all public libraries and consumer health collections."
—*Library Journal*

"A well-organized format with critical information and resources at your fingertips . . . educates the reader about the many issues that stand before people living with chronic conditions and provides answers and avenues for getting the best care possible."
—MSWorld, Inc. www.msworld.org

"A masterful job of presenting the multiple aspects of caregiving in a format that is both comprehensive and reader-friendly . . . important focus on physical aspects of giving care."
—Parkinson Report

"Almost any issue or question or need for resolution is most likely spoken of somewhere within the pages of this guide."
—*American Journal of Alzheimer's Disease*

"Physicians, family practitioners and geriatricians, and hospital social workers should be familiar with the book and recommend it to families of the elderly."
—Reviewers Choice, Home Care University

"An excellent guide on caregiving in the home. Home health professionals will find it to be a useful tool in teaching family caregivers."
—Five Star Rating, *Doody's Health Sciences Review Journal*

"Overall a beautifully designed book with very useful, practical information for caregivers."
—Judges from the Benjamin Franklin Awards

"Noteable here are the specifics. Where others focus on psychology alone, this gets down to the nitty gritty."
—*The Midwest Book Review*

"We use *The Comfort of Home*™ for the foundational text in our 40-hour Caregiver training. I believe it is the best on the market."
—Linda Young, Project Manager, College of the Desert

Part One: Getting Ready

Understanding Alzheimer's Disease

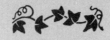

Understanding Alzheimer's Disease

*A*lthough changes in memory, such as forgetting names, are normal as people age, severe memory loss that interferes with daily life is not a normal part of aging. The loss of intellectual functions such as thinking, remembering, and reasoning is called dementia.

Memory Loss—Is It Just Forgetfulness or Is It Dementia?

A person with dementia will have symptoms that include short- and long-term memory loss, as well as difficulties learning new things, understanding abstract ideas (ideas that are not clearly spelled out), problem solving, concentrating, coordination, judgment, language, orientation (being aware of where you are), motor integration (muscles working together), and social skills.

There are over 70 possible causes of dementia. Alzheimer's disease (AD) is the most common form of dementia. Vascular dementia, which is caused by blood not flowing properly to the brain, accounts for about 20% of all cases of dementia. Dementia with Lewy Bodies accounts for another 20% of cases. Even rarer causes of chronic dementia include Huntington's disease, Pick's disease, AIDS, Lou Gehrig's disease, Creutzfeldt-Jacob disease, and multiple sclerosis. There are *reversible* causes of dementia, such as vitamin and hormone deficiencies, other medical illnesses, and emotional problems.

Some causes of dementia can be improved or corrected. A thorough evaluation is needed to figure out the reason for the memory loss. Anyone suspected of having dementia should have a full diagnostic evaluation to determine the cause of the symptoms. Teaching hospitals generally have a geriatric assessment center. Call your local Area Agency on Aging for the nearest diagnostic center.

What Is Alzheimer's Disease?

Alzheimer's disease causes changes in the brain that result in the sickness and death of neurons (nerve cells), brain atrophy (shrinkage), and an abnormal accumulation of toxic proteins [deposits known as neurofibrillary tangles and amyloid (*am-ah-loyd*) plaques].

Alzheimer's does not occur suddenly, like a stroke or heart attack. Alzheimer's disease progresses gradually over time. Damage to the brain takes place over many years, sometimes without being noticed, before symptoms become severe enough to cause concern.

When first described in 1906 AD was considered a rare illness. Today we know that Alzheimer's disease is the most common cause of dementia in older adults. The Alzheimer's Association estimates that more than 5 million people are living with Alzheimer's disease in the United States today. One in 10 families has a relative with Alzheimer's disease. The greatest risk factor for Alzheimer's is getting older: it has been estimated that about half the population over 85 is affected.

Checklist

WARNING SIGNS of Alzheimer's—Normal Aging vs Alzheimer's Disease

The Alzheimer's Association, the world leader in Alzheimer's research and support, has developed a checklist of common symptoms to help recognize the warning signs of Alzheimer's disease:

✓ **Memory loss**—*Forgetting recently learned information is one of the most common early signs of dementia. A person begins to forget more often and is unable to recall the information later.*

What's Normal Aging? Forgetting names or appointments occasionally.

✓ **Difficulty performing familiar tasks**—*People with dementia often find it hard to plan or complete everyday tasks. Individuals may lose track of the steps needed to prepare a meal, place a telephone call, or play a game.*

What's Normal Aging? Occasionally forgetting why you came into a room or what you planned to say.

✓ **Problems with language**—*People with Alzheimer's disease often forget simple words or substitute unusual words, making their speech or writing hard to understand. They may be unable to find the toothbrush, for example, and instead ask for "that thing for my mouth."*

What's Normal Aging? Sometimes having trouble finding the right word.

✓ **Disorientation to time and place**—*People with Alzheimer's disease can become lost in their own neighborhoods, forget where they are and how they got there, and not know how to get back home.*

What's Normal Aging? Forgetting the day of the week or where you were going.

Poor or decreased judgment—*Those with Alzheimer's may dress inappropriately, wearing several layers on a warm day or little clothing in the cold. They may show poor judgment about money, like giving away large sums to telemarketers.*

What's Normal Aging? Making a questionable or debatable decision from time to time.

Problems with abstract thinking—*Someone with Alzheimer's disease may have unusual difficulty performing complex mental tasks, like forgetting what numbers are and how they should be used.*

What's Normal Aging? Finding it challenging to balance a checkbook.

Misplacing things—*A person with Alzheimer's disease may put things in unusual places: an iron might go in the freezer or a wristwatch in the sugar bowl.*

What's Normal Aging? Misplacing keys or a wallet temporarily.

Changes in mood or behavior—*Someone with Alzheimer's disease may show rapid mood swings–from calm to tears to anger–for no apparent reason.*

What's Normal Aging? Occasionally feeling sad or moody.

Changes in personality—*The personalities of people with dementia can change dramatically. They may become extremely confused, suspicious, fearful, or dependent on a family member.*

What's Normal Aging? People's personalities do change somewhat with age.

Loss of initiative—*A person with Alzheimer's disease may become very passive, sitting in front of the TV for hours, sleeping more than usual, or not wanting to do usual activities.*

What's Normal Aging? Sometimes feeling weary of work or social obligations.

Source: © 2005 Alzheimer's Association. All rights reserved.
This is an official publication of the Alzheimer's Association but may be distributed by unaffiliated organizations or individuals. Such distribution does not constitute an endorsement of these parties or their activities by the Alzheimer's Association.

What Happens to the Brain?

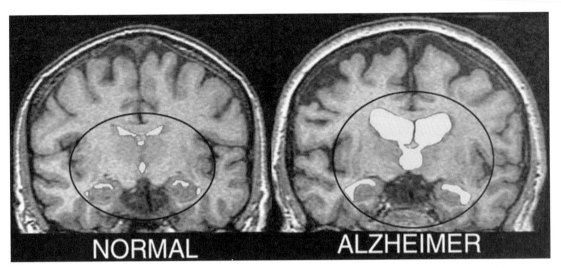

NORMAL   ALZHEIMER

White spaces in Alzheimer scan are places where brain cells have been destroyed.

Picture courtesy of Mony de Leon, NYU Alzheimer's Disease Center.

The brain is made up of nerve cells called neurons. They send messages to each other that make us able to think and act. With Alzheimer's disease, the buildup of protein deposits called amyloid plaques gathers in the spaces between the neurons and tangles form in the neurons. There are also changes in the chemical messengers that carry information from one neuron to another, preventing them from communicating with each other. The cells in certain areas of the brain deteriorate earlier than others, but eventually the whole brain is affected. As nerve cells die and the brain shrinks, a person's ability to function gradually declines.

Alzheimer's disease typically occurs in older adults. However, it may occur before age 65, in which case it is called "early onset." When it occurs in younger adults, the progression of the disease is often faster. The fact that it can sometimes occur in a younger adult makes it clear that AD is a disease, and not a necessary consequence of aging.

Why Get A Diagnostic Evaluation?

Sometimes fear of finding out the truth about their memory problems stops people from seeking a doctor's opinion (diagnosis), but a thorough check-up may identify a *treatable* condition. Even if the diagnosis confirms the presence of an illness that causes irreversible dementia, it may still be a relief to everyone concerned to finally learn the cause of the problem.

The advantage of getting an early diagnosis is the person with AD will be able to participate in making plans for the future. Also, you will learn—

- about resources and treatments to help you.
- what to expect from the person in your care.
- what will be expected of *you*, who are about to become a caregiver.

If you know what symptoms are likely to appear at each stage of the illness, you will be able to prepare for the best way to handle them, making the most of the person's remaining strengths and abilities.

Diagnosis

A good place to start the diagnostic process is with the person's primary doctor. The doctor may order screening tests and may give an initial diagnosis. Then the doctor may refer the person to a specialized center for memory evaluation, or to a neurologist (a nervous system specialist), geriatrician (a specialist in old age), or a psychiatrist for additional testing to be sure the diagnosis is correct.

Tip

The person in your care may resist going to the doctor for an evaluation of his memory problems. Perhaps it will help to tell the person that there is a physical reason for the doctor's visit, such as a blood pressure and cholesterol check-up for both of you. Or you may tell the person you want to have a memory evaluation yourself so that you can share the experience.

At good diagnostic centers, doctors can now determine whether a person has Alzheimer's disease with greater than 90% certainty after a thorough evaluation. An evaluation will include—

- Medical history

- Psychological tests

- Medical tests

- Physical examination

- Brain scans

- Information from the person with the illness and from someone who knows the patient well, who can describe changes that have occurred

Treatments and Medications

Currently, there is no medication that can stop or cure Alzheimer's disease. There are FDA-approved drugs available that can slow the progression of some of the symptoms and may offer modest improvements in memory and cognitive function in some patients. Certain antipsychotic and antiepileptic drugs, which are used for people with other conditions, can sometimes be prescribed to reduce agitation (nervousness) in the middle stages of Alzheimer's disease. But these and all medications need to be prescribed with caution. There are currently many efforts underway to find new treatments. Enrolling in a clinical trial of a medication may give you access to the newest kinds of treatment at no cost before they are widely available. Check with your local Alzheimer's Association or on the Internet at www.Clinical Trials.gov for the latest information.

NOTE At this time, the most effective treatment for Alzheimer's disease—more effective than any drug—is having a competent and *kind* caregiver. A caregiver who understands the illness, knows how to communicate with the person, creates a warm, safe home and offers interesting activities with love and encouragement.

Supporting Strengths and Abilities

Involvement in social and comfortably challenging activities may help slow the functional decline that comes with the illness. There are ways to make the most of the person's remaining strengths and reduce the disability caused by Alzheimer's disease. Just as it is for everyone, it is important to maintain the general health of a person with Alzheimer's disease. Proper nutrition, exercise, hearing, and vision aids and care of other illnesses can help the person function as well as possible (see *Health Care for the Person with Alzheimer's Disease*, p. 103).

> **NOTE** Care needs change over time. There are a few principles to always keep in mind:
>
> 1. The heart of care is the *relationship* between the caregiver and the care receiver.
>
> 2. Focus on the effort the ill person makes, and not the result.
>
> 3. Maintain the dignity and self-esteem of the person with Alzheimer's disease.

The Stages of Alzheimer's Disease

Symptoms don't occur in the same order in all people, and everyone with Alzheimer's disease does not get *all* of the symptoms. It is important to understand that the effects of Alzheimer's disease change over time. Your caregiving responsibilities will change as well. The following list of changes that usually occur at each stage is meant to give you a general idea of what will happen.

Early Stage—Common Changes in Mild AD

- The person appears physically the same and may handle casual conversations almost normally

- Forgets names

- May lose spark or zest for life and feel depressed

- May have difficulty starting activities

- Forgets events shortly after they happen

- May handle money unreliably

- Has difficulty learning new things and making new memories

- Has trouble finding words—may substitute or make up words that sound like or mean something like the forgotten word

- May talk less to avoid making mistakes
- Has a shorter attention span and less ability to stay with an activity
- May lose her way going to familiar places
- May resist change or new things
- Has trouble organizing and thinking logically
- Asks repetitive questions
- Withdraws, loses interest, is irritable, may seem less sensitive to others' feelings
- May get uncharacteristically angry when frustrated or tired
- Has difficulty making choices and decisions; for example, when asked what she wants to eat, says "I'll have what she is having"
- Takes longer to do routine chores and becomes upset if rushed or if something unexpected happens
- May forget to pay, pays too much, or forgets how to pay
- Forgets to eat, eats only one kind of food, or eats constantly
- Loses or misplaces things by hiding them in odd places or forgets where things go, such as putting clothes in the dishwasher
- Constantly checks, searches, or hoards things of no value

Middle Stage—Common Changes in Moderate AD

- Behavioral and psychological symptoms occur often
- Less concern for appearance and personal hygiene
- Sleep pattern changes

- Mixes up identity of people, such as thinking a son is a brother or that a wife is a stranger

- Poor judgment creates safety issues when left alone—may wander and be at risk of exposure, poisoning, falls, self-neglect, or exploitation

- Has trouble recognizing familiar people and possessions; may take things that belong to others

- Repeats stories, favorite words, statements, or movements—such as tearing tissues

- Has restless, repetitive movements in late afternoon or evening, such as pacing, trying doorknobs, fingering draperies

- Cannot organize thoughts or follow logical explanations

- Has trouble following written notes or completing tasks

- Makes up stories to fill in gaps in memory. For example might say, "Mama will come for me when she gets off work."

- May be able to read but may not understand the content

- Cannot formulate the correct response to a written request

- May accuse, threaten, curse, fidget or behave inappropriately, such as kicking, hitting, biting, screaming, or grabbing

- May forget traditional table manners

- May see, hear, smell, or taste things that are not there

- May accuse spouse of an affair or family members of stealing

- Naps frequently or awakens at night believing it is time to go to work

- Has more difficulty positioning the body to use the toilet or sit in a chair
- May be incontinent either all or some of the time
- May think mirror image is following him or television story is happening to her
- Needs help finding the toilet, using the shower, remembering to drink, and dressing for the weather or occasion
- Exhibits inappropriate sexual behavior, perhaps mistaking another individual for a spouse. Forgets what is private behavior, and may disrobe or masturbate in public (this behavior is very rare)

Late Stage—Common Changes in Severe AD

- Doesn't recognize herself or close family
- May pat or touch everything
- Speaks, but it is difficult or impossible to understand the content
- May become mute
- May refuse to eat, forgets to chew and swallow
- May choke on food
- Control of bowel and bladder is lost
- Forgets how to walk or is too unsteady or weak to stand alone
- May repetitively cry out
- Loses weight and skin becomes thin and tears easily
- May look uncomfortable or cry out when transferred or touched
- May develop contractures (tightening of the muscles) that cause pain when person is moved
- May have seizures, frequent infections, falls

- May groan, scream, or mumble loudly

- Sleeps more

- Becomes bedridden

- Needs total assistance for all activities of daily living

*Adapted from Gwyther, LP. (1985). *Care of Alzheimer's Patients: A Manual for Nursing Home Staff.*

We can only provide a rough idea of how long each stage will last, as there is a lot of difference among people. The mild stage of AD generally lasts about two years. The moderate stage can last four years. The severe stage can last seven or more years. The length of each stage depends on many factors, including the age of the person and the other illnesses the person has. There are several rating scales that are commonly used by health care professionals to determine the stage of Alzheimer's disease a person is in. The most widely used scales for measuring a person's mental and functional abilities are the Global Deterioration Scale (GDS), the Clinical Dementia Rating (CDR), and the Functional Assessment Staging (FAST) scale.

The Perspective of the Person with AD

Not all people with Alzheimer's disease respond to the diagnosis in the same way. Some seem not to react, some seem relieved, while others become depressed.

Those who do not *show* they care when given the diagnosis may actually be in denial. They brush off the changes that others can see or they may be so advanced in the disease that they do not understand the diagnosis.

NOTE It is not helpful to try to convince a person that he has a diagnosis of Alzheimer's disease if he denies it. It may be easier for him to accept being told he has a memory problem.

Others who accept their diagnosis may be painfully aware of the skills and abilities they are losing and become depressed. Supportive counseling and possibly medication may be helpful.

And then there are those who react to the diagnosis with relief that they *finally* have an explanation of their symptoms. They may then begin planning for the future and doing things they might otherwise have put off.

People in the early stage of AD may take comfort from interacting with others in their situation, either as members of a support group or by participating in Internet organizations, such as DASNI (Dementia Advocacy and Support Network International), a worldwide organization run by and for those diagnosed with dementia (see *Resources*, p. 19).

NOTE It is essential that family and professional caregivers focus on the remaining strengths of people with AD and encourage and support their ongoing participation in family and community life. Now that AD is often being diagnosed while people are still in its earliest stages, they are beginning to speak out on their own behalf and to seek supportive services. As a result, a fuller appreciation of the experience and perspective of the person with AD is developing. Family members and other care providers should welcome this. Try to understand their perspective and encourage them to participate in the discussion of their needs, care, and treatment.

The Effects on the Family

Alzheimer's disease affects not only the person with the illness, but the rest of the family as well. The family may need to reorganize and to create a care plan that will support all its members while coping with feelings of sadness, loss, and the fear of change. Plans that have been made and looked forward to may need to be changed or given up. New roles and skills may need to be developed. The symptoms can put a strain on relationships.

Family members responsible for the care of the person with Alzheimer's can become depressed. Young children can be frightened by the symptoms of Grandma or Grandpa. Tensions can develop about *who* will provide care, and *what kind* of care to provide. Therefore, family members should find information, counseling, and support.

Caregiving has positive aspects as well. Caregivers often describe positive feelings and experiences such as feeling more confident about themselves, proud that they have taken good care of the person with dementia, and grateful for all the help and kindness, and the wonderful people they have met. Caregiving has been described as a career and as a journey. The person with Alzheimer's disease can be ill for as long as twenty years. As a caregiving family member or friend, you need to prepare as best you can, accept support when it is offered, give yourself permission to make mistakes, and honor your life and that of the person with dementia.

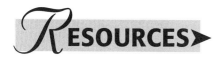

Alzheimer's Association
225 North Michigan Avenue
Fl. 17
Chicago, IL 60601
(312) 335-8700
24-hour Helpline (800) 272-3900
TDD (312) 335-8882
http://www.alz.org
Provides free literature and can refer you to the nearest local chapter that assists caregivers and family members and people with Alzheimer's disease.

Alzheimer's Disease Education and Referral Center
P.O. Box 8250
Silver Spring, MD 20907
(800) 438-4380
Fax (301) 495-3334
http://www.alzheimers.org/adear
Sponsored by the National Institute on Aging, this organization provides information and publications on Alzheimer's disease to caregivers and the public.

American Health Assistance Foundation
15825 Shady Grove Road
Suite 140
Rockville, MD 20850
(800) 437-AHAF (2423)
http://www.ahaf.org
Provides a variety of written materials on Alzheimer's disease.

Dementia Advocacy and Support Network International (DASNI)

http://www.dasninternational.org/

DASNI is a worldwide organization run by and for those diagnosed with dementia.

http://ClinicalTrials.gov

This Web site provides regularly updated information about federally and privately supported clinical research in human volunteers. ClinicalTrials.gov gives you information about a trial's purpose, who may participate, locations, and phone numbers for more details. The information provided on ClinicalTrials.gov should be used in conjunction with advice from health care professionals.

Publications

Alzheimer's Early Stages: First Steps for Family Friends and Caregivers by Daniel Kuhn, MSW; Alameda CA: Hunter House, 2003.

A Dignified Life: The Best Friends Approach to Alzheimer's Care: A Guide for Family Caregivers. By Virginia Bell and David Troxel; Deerfield Beach, FL: Health Communication Press, 2002.

Partial View: An Alzheimer's Journal, C. S., Henderson, & N. Andrews, N. Dallas, TX: Southern Methodist University, 1998.

The 36-hour Day: A Family Guide to Caring for Persons with Alzheimer Disease, Related Dementing Illnesses, and Memory Loss in Later Life by Nancy L. Mase, MA and Peter V. Rabins, MD; Baltimore, MD: Johns Hopkins University Press, 2006.

Video

The Family Guide to Understanding Alzheimer's Disease. LifeView Resources $99.95, five volume set. Available from www.comfortofhome.com.

Preparing the Home

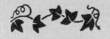

Preparing the Home

our goal in adapting the home for a person with Alzheimer's disease (AD) is to keep the surroundings as familiar as possible, while making the changes necessary to create a home that is calming, reassuring, safe, and supportive. This will make it possible for the person with dementia to be as independent as possible and for you to provide care as it is needed.

Creating a Safe Home Environment

Creating a safe home environment for a person with Alzheimer's disease requires changes that would be made for any older person, but you should also consider any physical or mental disabilities he or she has that are unique to Alzheimer's disease and try to plan ahead for future difficulties.

The environment should be suitable or right for the symptoms of the disease, which include—

- Memory loss
- Confusion about where he is
- Confusion about how to get to or find a particular room
- Decreased judgment
- Tendency to wander
- Poor impulse control
- Changes in vision, hearing, depth perception
- Sensitivity to changes in temperature

You can't predict every need that will come along. Alzheimer's disease symptoms get worse as time goes on. In the early stage it causes mostly thinking (cognitive) difficulties. Eventually it causes physical decline as well. In the late or severe stage, the loss of abilities such as walking has a major effect on how much care will be needed. Features of the home, such as steps and narrow bathroom doors, can become major obstacles to providing care.

While the behavior of the person in your care may sometimes seem highly unpredictable, and leave you feeling off balance and upset, you may feel more in control if you learn what to expect in the future because of the disease and make the changes to your home early on. This way you know you are getting as ready as you can for what will follow.

Not all changes to the home need to be made at once. Remember that it is difficult for a person with AD to adjust to changes in the environment. For this reason, it may be best to make some changes when the person is in the early stage of the illness and will have the easiest time getting used to them.

If you are making changes to a home in which you do not live, your parent's home, for example, be aware and sensitive to what these possessions mean to the elderly person and proceed with sensitivity. While sorting, you may come across an old childhood item of yours that your parents saved and you haven't thought about in years. The tug at your heart as you move it to the get-rid-of pile is a hint of the challenge and pain that is part of Alzheimer's care.

Some caregivers feel that so much is already being asked of them that to change a home that is familiar and pleasant is very distressing. Thoughts like, "I don't want my home to look like a hospital" are completely understandable. Each caregiver has to find her own way of dealing with this. Your dislike of adjusting to a raised toilet seat, for example, can give you insight into the adjustments a person with Alzheimer's needs to make just as the disease is slowly robbing him of the ability to have a say about those changes. Having compassion for the person with the illness will help you to plan for gradual changes to the home that will be needed as the disease progresses. Having an understanding of the disease will help you feel less resentment about them.

When the necessary changes are made, the home will be safer. The person with Alzheimer's disease will be able to function better and your job as a caregiver will be less physically and emotionally stressful. The chance of a fall, an accident, and frightening experiences such as having the person in your care wander away from home will be reduced. As you think about the safety you will gain, adapting the home may seem much more worthwhile. You may find that in the end you are pleased with the steps you have taken to improve the quality of life of the person with AD and the care you can provide.

Although the list of suggestions is long, only make those changes that are relevant to your situation. The fewer changes made to get the job done the better.

Safety, Safety, Safety

"In 2003, almost 13,000 people 65 and older died from a fall. Of those, 7,500 occurred in the home and 2,500 in a residental setting. . . . Among all age groups 'falls' ranked as the second leading cause of unintentional injury deaths in the United States. Of those who survive a fall, 20–30 percent will suffer debilitating injuries that affect them the rest of their lives" (Source: National Safety Council, Report on Injuries in America, 2003).

The main concern in any home is safety. Accidents can happen, but with a little planning can be prevented. Take a close look at the home where you will provide care.

As you plan for safety in the home, think about what you will need now and what you will need in the future. For example, furniture that works well for a 65-year-old may need to be changed or replaced later as the person loses strength. Your first concern is to make the home as safe as possible.

As you make changes to the home, don't forget your own comfort and ease. Making life easier for yourself means you will have more time to provide care or to rest. In the long run, this will improve the overall setting for care.

General Home Safety for the Person with Alzheimer's Disease

When caring for someone with Alzheimer's at home you are providing a chance for that person to remain in a familiar, comfortable environment where he can use his strengths and be encouraged to be as independent as possible for as long as possible. A safe, comfortable home can help a person with Alzheimer's feel more relaxed and less overwhelmed. Try to look at the world through the eyes of a person with AD and above all focus on preventing accidents, wandering away from home, and emotional upset. Ask a friend or relative to look at it with you to make sure you have not overlooked any hazards.

Safety

For the safest home, follow as many of these steps as possible:

• Remove any furniture that is not needed.

• Place the remaining furniture so that there is enough space for a walker or wheelchair. This will avoid the need for an elderly or disabled person to move around coffee tables and other barriers. Move any low tables that are in the way.

- Once the person in your care has gotten used to where the furniture is, do not change it.

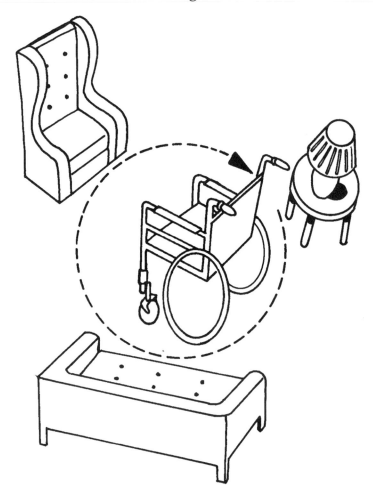

▶ *To accommodate a wheelchair, arrange furniture 5¹/₂ feet apart.*

- Make sure furniture will not move if it is leaned on.

- Make sure the armrests of a favorite chair are long enough to help the person get up and down.

- Add cushioning to sharp corners on furniture, cabinets, and vanities.

- Keep a telephone and flashlight where they are easily available.

- Keep power tools and other dangerous equipment where they are not accessible to the person with AD.

- Remove clutter.

- Remove scatter rugs, which can cause trips and falls.

- Place protective screens in front of fireplaces.

- Cover exposed hot-water pipes.

- Have a carpenter install railings in places where a person might need extra support. (Using a carpenter can ensure that railings can bear a person's full weight and will not give way.) It is worthwhile to consult with an expert, such as a physical or occupational therapist, for help in placing grab bars and safety rails. If they are not in the right position or securely attached they will not lend the support they are intended to provide. The screws MUST go into the wall studs.

- Plan for extra outdoor lighting for good nighttime visibility, especially on stairs and walkways.

- If the person with dementia is incontinent, use fabric pads that blend with the upholstery. These are available in many colors and are machine washable. These may not cause the embarrassment that regular pads can.

- Make chair seats 20″ high. (Wood blocks or a wooden platform can be placed under large, heavy furniture to raise it to this level.)

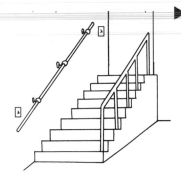

▲ *Always provide railings along stairways. When possible, extend the handrail past the bottom and top step.*

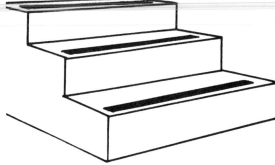

▶*Place nonskid tape on the edges of steps.*

- Place masking or colored tape on glass doors and picture windows.

- Use automatic night-lights in the rooms used by the person in your care.

- Clear fire-escape routes.

- Provide smoke alarms on every floor and outside every bedroom.

- Place a fire extinguisher in the kitchen.

- Think about using monitors and intercoms.

- Place nonskid tape on the edges of stairs (and consider painting the edge of the first and last step a different color from the floor to help with depth perception).

▶ *Thresholds should be fixed in such a way to avoid tripping. If possible, they should be beveled, or slanted and gradual, not angled.*

No ⟶ ◀ Yes

▶ *Put in nonskid flooring or use nonskid floor waxes.*

▼ *Tack or tape down loose carpets.*

- Install a sturdy gate with a lock on any dangerous stairs. Gate must be higher than the person with AD's waist. Baby gates are dangerous as people may try to climb over them.

- It is easier to walk on thin-pile carpet than on thick pile. Avoid busy patterns.

- Be sure stairs have even surfaces with no metal strips or rubber mats to cause tripping.

- Remove all hazards that might lead to tripping.

- Adjust or remove rapidly closing doors.

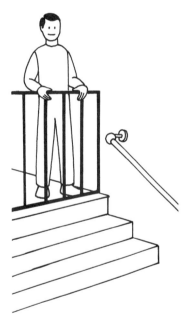

▲ *A safety gate at the top of stairs can prevent falls.*

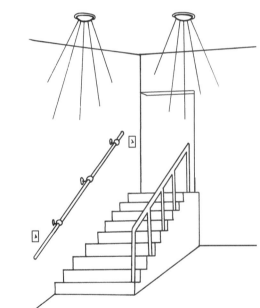

▲ *Be sure steps are well lighted with light switches at both the top and bottom of the stairs.*

- Cover exposed hot-water pipes.

- Provide enough no-glare lighting—indirect is best.

- Place light switches next to room entrances so the lights can be turned on before entering a room. Consider "clap-on" lamps beside the bed.

- Use 100- to 200–watt lightbulbs for close-up activities (but make sure lamps can handle the extra wattage).

- For those who tend to wander, create a safe path through the home for a "wander loop."

- Put reflector tape on furniture and sharp corners.

- Use reflector tape to create a path to follow from the bedroom to the bathroom at night.

- Cover radiators with radiator guards.

- Use child-proof plugs in all electrical outlets.

- Lock the cellar and garage doors; hide the garage remote control.

- Lock liquor cabinets.

- Remove or lock up all poisonous household items. Colorful cleaning products may be mistaken for food.

- Remove all sharp items.

- Remove poisonous plants from the house and yard.

- Install safety latches/locks on the doors and fenced/gated exteriors. Install alarms on the doors.

- Rid the home of firearms or store them in a locked cabinet, with the bullets in a separate locked cabinet.

- Cover smooth or shiny surfaces to reduce glare, which upsets or confuses the person with Alzheimer's.

- Eliminate shadows by creating a uniform level of light with uplights that reflect off the ceiling. (Ask a lighting store for a lamp that doesn't cast shadows.)

- Cover or remove mirrors if they are upsetting to the person with AD, who may not recognize himself.

- Store car keys in a locked container; ask a mechanic to disable the car so you can still use it but the person with AD cannot.

 An 85-year-old needs about three times the amount of light a 15-year-old needs to see the same thing. Contrasting colors play a big part in seeing well. As much as possible, the color of furniture, toilet seats, counters, etc., should be different from the floor color.

 A person with Alzheimer's disease may not understand how to use power-assisted devices, and thus they may create more danger than benefit.

 Apartment dwellers should hang a personalized item on the front door to help the person with AD recognize his apartment.

Comfort and Convenience

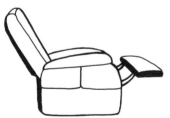

- For persons who are frail or wheelchair-bound, put in automatic door openers.
- For a person with a wheelchair or a walker, allow at least 18–24″ clearance from the door on landings.
- Plan to leave enough space (a minimum of 32″ clear) for moving a hospital bed and wheelchair through doorways.

▲ *Think about getting a recliner that doesn't have a power-assist feature, but works manually.*

▶ *Install entry ramps. Rails can be added for more safety.*

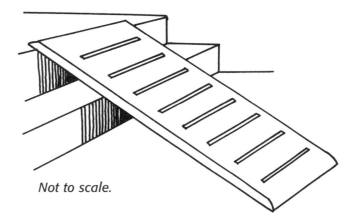

Not to scale.

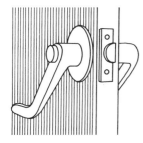

▲ *Lever handle*

- To widen doorways, remove the molding and replace regular door hinges with offset hinges. Whenever possible, remove doors.

- Put lever-type handles on all doors.

- If a person who is disabled must be moved from one story to another, install a stair elevator.

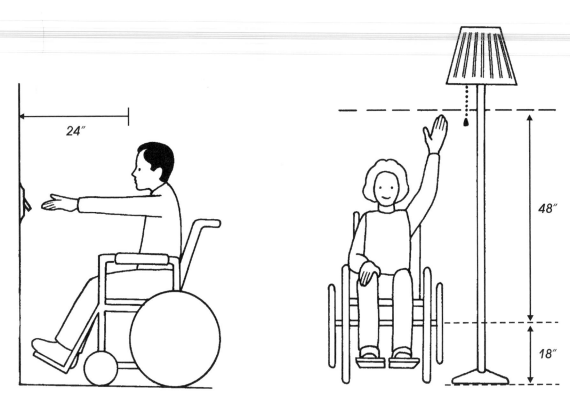

▲ *A person can reach forward about 24" from a seated position. Between 18" and 48" from the floor is the ideal position for light switches, telephones, and mailboxes.*

- Place fragile items of monetary or sentimental value where they cannot be accidentally broken.

- Lock important documents out of reach.

- Try to have windows low enough to look out when sitting; however, intall guards to prevent them from being opened more than 3 inches.

- Choose wall colors that are soothing and are favorites of the person in your care.

Prepare in Advance for Emergencies

- Keep emergency numbers near every telephone.
- If possible, install a carbon monoxide (CO) detector that sounds an alarm when dangerous levels of CO are reached. Call the American Lung Association, (800) LUNG USA, for details.
- Work out an emergency escape plan in case of fire.

Note: Make a list of vital care information such as the person's doctor, medications, and insurance information. Put it in plain sight—usually on the refrigerator—for emergency workers or for a new caregiver.

Now let's look at specific rooms and how you can make them safer. Let's start with the bathroom.

The Bathroom

Take great care when setting up the bathroom. With some forethought potential dangers can be avoided.

Safety

- It is difficult to get in and out of a tub enclosed with glass doors. A shower curtain may make life simpler.
- Nonskid decals will make the tub less slippery and may even provide a useful distraction at bath time.
- When the person in your care is no longer able to stand firmly and confidently in the shower, a shower bench can provide safety and security in the tub as well as the shower.
- Clear out or lock the medicine chest and the cabinet under the sink where poisonous substances have been kept.

- If the person with Alzheimer's disease shaves, a cordless rechargeable electric razor is safest. A safety razor should only be used with supervision.

- A raised toilet seat that has hand rails will make it easier to get up and down. Replace an uncomfortable hard toilet seat with a soft cushiony one.

- A shut-off mechanism and a mechanism to control water temperature in sink, tub, and shower will prevent accidental flooding and burns.

▶ *Install grab bars beside the toilet, along the edge of the sink, and in the tub and shower according to the needs of each person.*

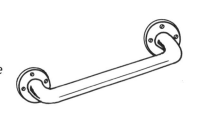

▶ *Five-inch door pulls or utility handles can be put on door frames and window sills.*

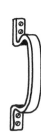

- Put screens over open drains

- Put wastebaskets out of sight. (Otherwise, a person with Alzheimer's may urinate in them or remove things from them.)

- Have no electrical cords dangling near the washbasin.

- Install an automatic hot and cold water mixer.

- If possible, have the toilet seat and washbasin in a contrasting color to the floor.

- Cover a sharp edges with rubber cushioning.

- Put lights in the medicine cabinets so mistakes are not made when giving medicine. People with AD should not be taking medications themselves.

- Remove locks on bathroom doors.

- Use nonskid safety strips or a nonslip bath mat in the tub or shower.

- Think about putting a grab rail on the edge of the vanity. (Do not use a towel bar.)

- Remove glass shower doors or replace them with unbreakable plastic or a shower curtain.

- Use only electrical appliances with a ground fault interrupted (GFI) feature.

- Install GFI electrical outlets.

- Set the hot water thermostat below 120° F.

- Use faucets that mix hot and cold water, or paint hot water knobs/faucets red.

- Insulate (cover) hot water pipes to prevent burns.

Comfort and Convenience

- People beyond the early stage of Alzheimer's disease should not be left alone in the bathroom. They may stuff the toilet with paper and cause a flood.

- If possible, the bathroom should be in a straight path from the bedroom of the person in your care.

- Put in a ceiling heat lamp.

- Provide soap-on-a-rope or put a bar of soap in the toe of a nylon stocking and tie it to the grab bar.

- Place toilet paper within easy reach.

- Try to provide enough space for two people at the bathroom sink.

- If possible, have the sink 32"–34" from the floor.

- Use levers instead of handles on faucets.

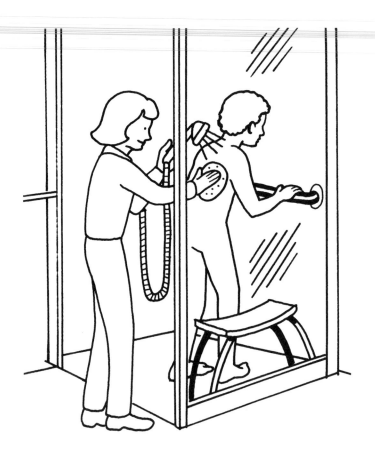

◀ *If possible, have a shower stall that is large enough for two people. Use a hand-held shower head with a very long hose and adjustable jet stream. Put a tub seat or bench in the shower stall.*

The Kitchen

The kitchen is filled with potential trouble spots. A person who is used to cooking may want to continue to do so but forget to turn off the flame when the food is done, may make the flame too high, or may not position pots safely on the stove top. At first, simply keeping close watch may be enough to reduce these risks. In time, as the disease progresses, it may be necessary to remove the knobs from the stove or to cover them so the person in your care will not notice them.

The microwave can be a mixed blessing. While it heats food quickly, the food can become too hot and the person with AD may use the wrong type of container and cause a fire. It may best be left unplugged with the plug out of sight.

People with AD sometimes put items in the refrigerator that do not belong there, such as a purse. They may also not be able to tell the difference between fresh food and rotten food or even food that needs to be cooked before it is eaten, such as raw hamburger. It may seem extreme to lock the refrigerator, but it might become necessary.

Safety

The following suggestions will make your kitchen a safer place for the person in your care:

- Remove spices or medicines from the counter tops and keep cleaning supplies in a locked place.

- Remove scissors and knives from counter tops and drawers. A person with AD may hurt himself or others with these dangerous items.

Tip

Put your favorite utensils in a place the person with Alzheimer's is not likely to find and move them. If you want to cook without interruptions, cook when he is sleeping or at day care. You will become as creative a caregiver as you are a cook.

- Remove all items that cause confusion.
- Disguise the garbage disposal switches.
- Put all the garbage out of sight.
- Put labels on the cabinets.
- Install a shut-off valve (for a gas stove) or a circuit breaker for an electric stove so you can disable it when you leave the kitchen.

- Remove burner knobs and tape the stems or install knob covers.

- Use a lock-out switch on the electric range so it can't be turned on except by you.

- Use an aluminum cover over the top of the stove, or use burner covers.

- Replace the pilot on a gas stove with an electric starter.

- Lock the oven door.

- Use safety latches on doors and cabinets.

- Install gates, door, or dutch doors so the kitchen can be closed off but you can still see and be seen.

- Install an automatic turn-off on the faucet.

- Install a governor on the hot water faucet (or turn down the valve under the sink) to control the amount of water that can be used.

- For a faucet spout that swings outside the sink itself, install a brace that keeps water in the sink at all times.

- Hide or get rid of dangerous small appliances.

- Turn off appliances by unplugging them, turning off circuit breakers, or removing fuses.

- Install smoke detectors (but not near the stove).

- Use an electric teakettle that has an automatic shutoff.

- Use a single-lever faucet that can balance water temperature.

- Provide an area away from the knife drawer and the stove where the person in your care can help prepare food.

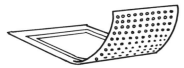

 Cover the floor with a nonslip surface or use a nonskid mat near the sink, where it may be wet.

- Ask the gas company to modify your stove to provide a gas odor that is strong enough to alert you if the pilot light goes out.

- Provide a step stool, never a chair, to reach high shelves.

Tip HELPING THE PERSON WITH ALZHEIMER'S COPE WITH MEMORY PROBLEMS

Here are some everyday steps that can be taken to help out.

- Colored paper or a picture of the toilet can be taped on bathroom door.

- Drawers, cabinets, and refrigerators can be labeled to show what's inside.

- Objects can be in contrasting colors so they stand out.

- Notes can be placed in plain sight as reminders of things the person in your care should do.

The Bedroom

Guard rails on the bed may sometimes be helpful supports when getting in and out of bed, but may also add to the risk of falls if the person attempts to climb over them. Consult with a physical therapist about the best way to use them, if at all, for the person in your care. A bed cane may turn out to be a safer alternative. It can offer support and increase balance. It is like a grab bar, with a wooden base that fits between the mattress and the box spring.

Night lights should be placed so that a person can find his way from the bedroom to the bathroom. Consider "clamp-on" lamps attached to the bed or wall lamps, which are less likely to fall over and cause a fire than lamps on a night table. Check for types that do not get hot.

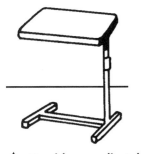

▲ *Provide an adjustable over-the-bed table like the ones used to serve meals in hospital rooms.*

- Place an alarm mat at the side of the bed, use an infrared sensor beam for sounding an alarm when a person crosses it, or attach a monitor to clothing.

- For anyone who is a wanderer, lower the bed height by removing casters, box springs, or legs; place the dresser at the end of the bed.

- Put in a monitor to listen to activity in the room of the person in your care. (Most are inexpensive and are portable.)

- Make the bedroom bright and cheerful.

- Make sure enough heat (65° F at night) and fresh air are available.

- Provide a firm mattress.

- Provide TV and radio.

- Think about having a fish tank for fun and relaxation. Be sure it is secure and the person in your care cannot knock it over by accident.

- Use throwaway pads to protect furniture.

- Install blinds or shades that darken the room.

- Place closet rods 48″ from the floor.

- Provide a chair for dressing.

- Keep a flashlight at the bedside table.

- Provide a bedside commode with a 4″ foam pad on the seat for comfort.

- Hang a bulletin board with pictures of family and friends where it can be easily seen.

- Provide a sturdy chair or table next to the bed for help getting in and out of bed.

- Make the bed 22″ high and place it securely against a wall. Or use lockable wheels. This will allow the person to get up and down safely.

- Use blocks to raise a bed's height, but be sure to make them steady so they don't move.

▶ *Bedside commode and bed with trapeze bar.*

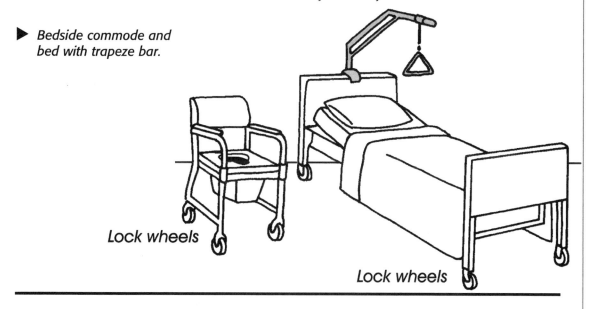

Lock wheels

Lock wheels

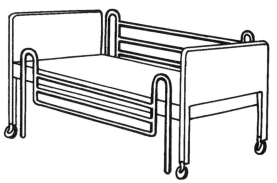

▲ *A hospital bed can make providing care easier, and make the person with AD more comfortable, as you can raise the back and foot without having to lift the person.*

Outdoor Areas

Safe outdoor areas are important, especially for those who are confused and are mobile. Safety features should include the following:

- ramps for access on ground that is not level or even
- a deck with a sturdy railing
- outside doors locked or alarmed
- a key hidden outside
- enough light to see walkway hazards at night
- nonslip step surfaces in good repair
- stair handrails fastened to their fittings
- step edges marked with reflective paint
- a hedge or fence around the yard and dangerous areas like pools or streams

In addition, unplug or remove power tools.

Doors, Windows, and Steps

Because a person with AD may want to leave the house on his own you may—

- Install an electric eye device that rings when someone goes out of the house.
- Put a lock close to the floor where he hopefully will not notice it.
- Use a cover over the door knob that will make it difficult to grasp and open.
- Put decals on the door that make it look like something else so that a person will not notice it. Lock sliding doors.

- Install window guards.
- Consider installing a keypad lock that requires the user to enter a code for the door to open.

 Medicare will pay for such equipment as a hospital bed, if it is prescribed by a doctor. Private insurance may also cover some of these items.

 GETTING ORGANIZED
Keep supplies together that are used often and keep a list of supplies so you can easily replace them.

 Be prepared for emergencies. Have on hand a flashlight, a battery-run radio, a battery-run clock, fresh batteries, extra blankets, candles with holders, matches, and a manual can opener.

Medical Equipment

Based on the stage of dementia and other illnesses that may handicap the person, you may need to have special equipment for different rooms in the house, as well as equipment to increase the person's ability to get around.

Equipment for the Bedroom

The equipment you need to have depends on the person's medical condition. This equipment might include some of the items listed below.

- **alternating pressure mattress**—reduces pressure on skin tissue

- **egg-carton pad**—a foam mattress pad shaped like the bottom of an egg carton that reduces pressure and improves air circulation

- **trapeze bar**—provides support and a secure hand-hold while changing positions

- **transfer board**—a smooth board for independent or assisted transfer from bed to wheelchair, toilet, or portable commode. This may be difficult for a person with AD, as he will have to follow instructions for it to be useful.

- **mechanical or electric lift chair**—for help getting up from a chair

- **urinal and bedpan**—for toileting in the bed. Note: It is very hard to cue a person with AD to use these.

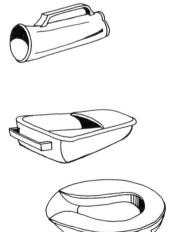

▲ *Urinal and bedpans*

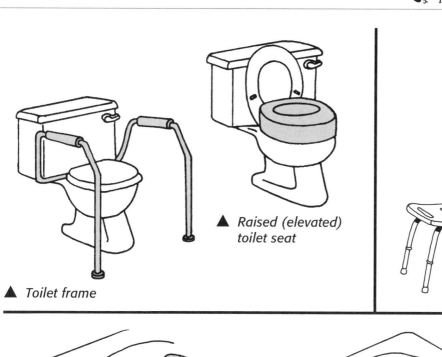

▲ Raised (elevated)
toilet seat

▲ Toilet frame

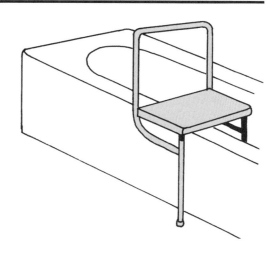

▲ Bath benches

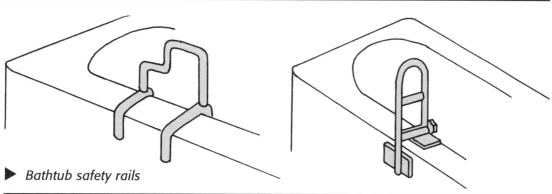

▶ Bathtub safety rails

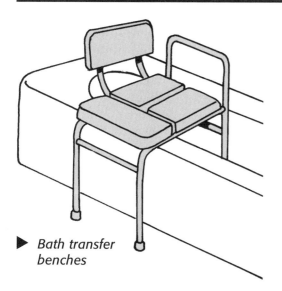

▶ Bath transfer
benches

Equipment for the Bathroom

The equipment you will need depends on the person's needs. You should consider providing the following:

- **commode aid**—a device that acts as an elevated toilet seat when used with a splash guard, or as a commode when used with a pail

- **toilet frame**—a free-standing unit that fits over the toilet and provides supports on either side for ease in getting up and down

- **grab bars for tub and shower**—properly installed wall-mounted safety bars that hold a person's weight

- **safety mat and strips**—rough vinyl strips that stick to the bottom of the tub and shower to prevent slipping

- **hand-held shower hose**—a movable shower hose and head that allows the water to be directed to all parts of the body

- **bath bench**—aid for a person who has difficulty sitting down in or getting up from the bottom of the tub

- **bath transfer bench**—a bench that goes across the side of the tub and allows a person to get out of the tub easily

- **bathtub safety rails**—support for getting in and out of the tub

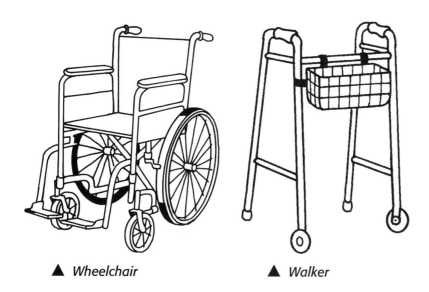

▲ *Wheelchair* ▲ *Walker*

Mobility Aids

You, as the caregiver, will have to learn how to teach the person in your care how to use some of these assistive devices. Some health care professionals believe, incorrectly, that a person with dementia cannot be taught. With patience and repeated instruction people with dementia can learn to use many of them. The person in your care can learn to use a walker, for example, even though he has never used one prior to developing AD. There is a lot to be lost by not trying, as immobility dramatically alters quality of life and physical health for the person with AD and makes caregiving more difficult.

Normally, physical therapists teach people to use these mobility aids. You may have to be an advocate for physical rehabilitation for a person with dementia. You should participate in the rehabilitation so you can learn how to help the person in your care maintain the routines.

Mobility aids include devices that help a person move around without help. They also help the caregiver transfer the person in and out of bed and from bed to a chair.

They include—

- a wheelchair with padding and removable arms

- a walker to help maintain balance and provide some support

- crutches when weight cannot be put on one leg or foot

- a cane to provide light weight-bearing support

- a transfer board (9" x 24") for moving someone in and out of bed

- a gait/transfer belt

▼ *Canes*

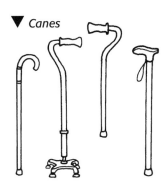

Wheelchair Requirements

Proper fit, as determined by a physical therapist.

- safety
- durability
- ease of repair
- attractive appearance

- comfort
- ease of handling
- cushions

USING CANES

Attach Velcro® to the top of a cane and a piece of Velcro® to counters and bedside tables to keep the cane from falling when not in use.

Wheelchair Attachments

- a brake lever extension on the handle

- elevated leg rests and removable footrests

- armrests that can be taken off

Some states have lemon laws that cover wheelchairs and other assistive devices. If you think there is something wrong with the equipment you have bought and you want to find out if it qualifies as a lemon, call the Attorney General's office in your state. They may be able to help you in getting a replacement or a refund.

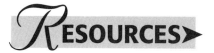

AARP
601 E Street, NW
Washington, DC 20049
(800) 424-3410
www.aarp.org
Call or write for the booklet, The Do-Able, Renewable Home. *Members can receive one copy at no charge.*

AbilityHub
www.abilityhub.com
Assistive technology for people who have difficulty operating a computer.

Adaptive Environments Center Inc.
374 Congress Street, Suite 301
Boston, MA 02210
(617) 695-1225 (v/tty); Fax (617) 482-8099
www.adaptiveenvironments.org
E-mail: info@adaptiveenvironments.org

Alliance for Technology Access
www.ataccess.org
A network of community-based resource centers, developers, vendors, and associates dedicated to providing information and support services to children and adults with disabilities, and increasing their use of standard, assistive, and information technologies. You can order their book Computer Resources for People with Disabilities *online.*

The Alzheimer's Store
(800) 752-3238
www.alzstore.com
Caregiving products designed to make caregiving and living with AD as easy as possible.

American Occupational Therapy Association (AOTA)
4720 Montgomery Lane
P.O. Box 31220
Bethesda, MD 20824-1220
(301) 652-2682; Fax (301) 652-7711
www.aota.org
Provides consumer publications.

Area Agency on Aging
Your local Area Agency on Aging provides home safety resources.

Center for Universal Design
North Carolina State University
Box 8613
Raleigh, NC 27695-8613
(800) 647-6777; (919) 515-3082 (V/TTY)
Fax: (919) 515-3023
www.design.ncsu.edu\cud
E-mail: cud@ncsu.edu
Established by the National Institute on Disability and Rehabilitation Research (NIDRR) to improve the quality and availability of housing for people with disabilities. Services include information, referral service, training and education, technical design assistance, and publications.

Hill-Rom
(800) 445-3730
www.hillrom.com
Provides a complete line of custom hospital beds, mattresses, furniture, and more for care at home.

Medic Alert®
(800) 432-5378
Offers critically important medical facts about the emblem wearer's condition to emergency personnel 24 hours a day.

Metropolitan Center for Independent Living, Inc. (MCIL)
1600 University Avenue West, Suite 16
St. Paul, MN 55104-3825
(651) 603-2029
www.wheelchairramp.org
E-mail: jimwi@mcil-mn.org
Web site features How to Build Wheelchair Ramps for Homes, *an online manual for the design and construction of wheelchair ramps.*

National Institute for Rehabilitation Engineering
P.O. Box 1088
Hewett, NJ 07421
(800) 736-2216; (973) 853-6585 Fax (928) 832-2894
www.theoffice.net/nire
E-mail: nire@theoffice.net

Paralyzed Veterans of America
801 18th Street NW
Washington, DC 20006-3517
(800) 424-8200
www.pva.org
Not just for veterans, not just for paralysis. Ask for the Architecture Program.

Radio Shack
Carries a variety of alerting devices in stores nationwide. Check your phonebook for store near you.

Sammons-Preston
Bolingbrook, IL
(800) 323-5547
Provider of rehabilitation equipment.

SCAN Medical
34 Sullivan Road, Unit 32
North Billerica, MA 01862
(888) 854-4687
info@scanmedical.com
www.scanmedical.com
SCAN Medical's manual-transfer devices are for people with impaired mobility. The products are of great help and assistance to caregivers to avoid back strain and to make normally difficult tasks easier.

Sears Home Health Care Catalogue
(800) 326-1750 for customer service
To place an order or find a Sears store near you.

SpeciaLiving Magazine
www.specialiving.com
Online info and store for accessible housing, special products, such as ramps, bathing systems, urinary devices, lifts.

Publications

The Complete Guide to Alzheimer's-Proofing Your Home by Mark Warner and Ellen Warner, Purdue University Press; revised edition, 2000.
This extremely useful guide deals with both interior and exterior spaces and shows how to create a home environment for Alzheimer's and related dementia; provides an exhaustive directory of manufacturers to locate the latest products for home health care.

For **medical alarms**, consult the phone book or contact your local hospital's long-term care or senior services division.

Check with local police to find out if they manage a **Senior Locks Program**. This program can install deadbolt locks and other security devices for homeowners 55 and older who meet federal income guidelines.

If you don't have access to the Internet, ask your local library to help you locate a Web site.

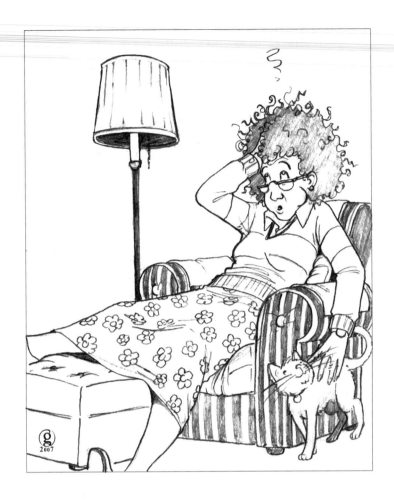

A good laugh and a long sleep are the two best cures.

—*Irish Proverb*

Hiring and Paying for Care

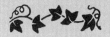

Hiring and Paying for Care

Hiring Paid Help

It may seem to you as though taking care of a person with Alzheimer's disease requires a never-ending series of decisions. One of the most sensitive decisions is whether you should hire someone to provide all or some of the care. This becomes complicated by the fact that the person with AD may say he does not see the need for more care, or may not want to be taken care of by a stranger. The family caregiver may also feel uncomfortable about hiring an outsider to provide care that he or she was previously giving. A variety of feelings, ranging from guilt to mistrust, together with practical issues such as finding the right person and figuring out how to pay for the service, further complicate taking this step. Your family may have differing perspectives about what care is needed and who should provide it. However, as the disease progresses it is almost always necessary for more than one person to take care of the person with AD and if family resources are not available, ultimately a professional caregiver will be needed at least some of the time.

If you belong to a support group you may have heard others talk about their emotional reactions to finding and working with paid help and bringing another person into their homes. The local chapter of the Alzheimer's Association or a counselor may be able to help you work out a care plan with which you feel comfortable.

When Will You Need Home Care Services?

There is no rule about when to seek home care. Typically home care services are needed when the person is in the moderate stage of AD, and can no longer be safely left alone and needs considerable hands-on care. However, you may need to hire someone to help with caring for the person with AD, even in the early stage of the illness if he or you have physical disabilities or he lives alone.

The severity of dementia may increase because of an illness or hospitalization, and the person may return to a higher level of functioning after recuperating. Sometimes the caregiver gets sick, or there are other demands on the caregiver's time and energy that make it necessary to hire help. In these cases the need for extra help may only be temporary.

Tip Keep in mind that even the Lone Ranger had a sidekick. You cannot do everything yourself.

What Kind of Help Can Others Offer?

Home care services can provide relief from caregiving, or additional support. A home care worker, sometimes called an aide, can be a friendly companion and take the ill person on walks or to a senior center. He or she can help with cooking, cleaning, and shopping as well as personal care such as bathing, dressing, and toileting. The aide can stay with the person with AD so that the caregiver can take care of other responsibilities, keep appointments, do errands, visit with friends, go to the gym, or just take a break from caregiving. It may take time and effort to find the right person, but when you do, you may find that you are more relaxed and feel more positive about your role as a caregiver.

Choosing a Home Care Worker

Before you hire someone, try to get a clear idea of what you would want them to do and the number of hours of work involved. It will cause problems if you do not express your expectations and agree on a plan. Also be sure to provide a good picture of the person who needs care—not only the physical care needs but also some history and the kinds of things the person likes to do. Try to match the potential home care worker to the interests and abilities and temperament of the person with AD. Remember: Care is about relationships and you want to make the best match you can.

NOTE ▷ It is essential that the person you hire understands the effects of Alzheimer's disease and how to communicate with and provide care for a person with this illness.

Working Together with the Person You Have Hired

Once you have hired someone, familiarize the aide with the home, the schedule, the person's taste in food and any other details that will help her to be appropriately responsive to the person she is caring for. Be sure that she has emergency contact information and understands the protocol. A copy of the Profile of the Person with Memory Impairment (see pp. 62–66) should be given to the aide.

It may help the person in your care to accept the new caregiver if you tell him that the aide is there to help *you*. Do not suggest in any way that it is because he or she is too much trouble for *you*. You too will have to learn to trust the person you have hired and to accept that she may not do things exactly as you would. She may do them differently but well enough. Encourage the aide to ask questions. In time, the person you have hired will understand the needs of the person she is caring for, and everyone will feel more comfortable. However, if you get the feeling that the person is not right, don't be afraid to make a change. Sometimes it takes some trial and error to find the right person.

NOTE At first, you may feel uneasy about leaving the aide alone with the person you have cared for. This is natural. And don't be surprised if you are not sure what to do with the free time you have worked so hard to create for yourself. This too is natural.

Caregivers who have been reluctant to hire a stranger to care for a family member often find that a warm and caring relationship develops that goes beyond everybody's expectations.

Photocopy form for your own personal use or visit
http://comfortofhome.com/Profile.pdf to download.

PROFILE OF A PERSON WITH MEMORY IMPAIRMENT

This profile describes the special needs of a person with Memory impairment. Its purpose is to help someone who does not know this person to understand how to take care of him or her. The profile describes how Memory impairment affects the way this person behaves, the areas in which s/he needs help, and how to calm and comfort him or her. It also includes a list of current medications and allergies. It can be used at home, in the hospital or physician's office, and anywhere else special care and knowledge of this person are required.

Date form completed_____
Mo/Da/Yr

Profile of _____**Date of Birth**_____
 First name   *Last name*   *Mo/Da/Yr*

Social Security #_____Medicare #_____

Medicaid #_____Other Medical Insurance_____

1. Primary contact_____
 First name   *Last name*

Telephone numbers *(home)*_____*(work)* _____

Other contact numbers_____
 (Specify: Cell, Voice Mail, Beeper, etc.)

Relationship of the person with memory impairment

_____Husband   _____Wife   _____Son   _____Daughter   _____Son-in-Law

_____Daughter-in-Law   _____Brother   _____Sister   _____Partner

Other *(specify)*_____

2. The person with memory impairment lives . . .

_____With primary caregiver   _____With another family member

_____Alone at home   _____In a nursing home

_____With primary caregiver and   _____With another family member
 paid caregiver   and paid caregiver

_____At home with paid caregiver   _____In an assisted-living facility

_____Other *(specify)*_____

Reprinted with permission from *The Alzheimer's Health Care Handbook: How to Get the Best Medical Care for Your Relative with Alzheimer's Disease, in and out of the Hospital,* by Mary S. Mittelman, DrPH and Cynthia Epstein, LCSW, 2002 Marlowe & Co, New York, Copyright 2002, 2003 by Mary S. Mittelman, DrPH.

3. Additional contacts

(1)_____ Relationship_____
    First name   *Last name*

Telephone number *(home)*_____*(work)*_____*(other)*_____
                                            (Specify: Cell, Voice Mail, Beeper, etc.)

(2)_____ Relationship_____
    First name   *Last name*

Telephone number *(home)*_____*(work)*_____*(other)*_____
                                            (Specify: Cell, Voice Mail, Beeper, etc.)

4. Person preparing this profile *(if not primary contact)*

_____ Relationship_____
    First name   *Last name*

Telephone number *(home)*_____*(work)*_____*(other)*_____
                                            (Specify: Cell, Voice Mail, Beeper, etc.)

5. Name of physician _____
               First name   *Last name*

Address_____ Telephone Number_____

Hospital affiliation_____

6. Hospital to which the person with memory impairment should be taken in an emergency

_____

7. Information that will help people care for the person with memory impairment

Does this person speak and understand English?   Yes No Don't know

If not, what language(s) does he or she speak? _____

Does this person...	Always	Sometimes	Never	Don't Know
understand where he or she is?				
answer questions accurately?				
follow instructions?				
remember what he or she is told?				
tell others what he or she needs?				
tell others when he or she is in pain?				
use the telephone without help?				

Does he or she...	Always	Sometimes	Never	Don't Know
normally use a hearing aid?				
use eyeglasses?				
have dentures?				

	Always	Sometimes	Never	Don't Know
Does this person normally need help feeding him or herself?				
If yes, does he or she need. . . food cut in pieces?				
to be helped to eat?				
to be fed by someone else?				

	Always	Sometimes	Never	Don't Know
Does he or she need help with toileting?				
If yes, does this person . . . indicate that he or she needs to go to the bathroom?				
need help finding the bathroom?				
need supervision while in the bathroom?				
need help with incontinence products?				
Is this person incontinent of urine?				
incontinent of feces?				

Does he or she need help ..	Always	Sometimes	Never	Don't Know
with personal hygiene (bathing, shampooing, brushing teeth, etc.?)				
with dressing?				
getting out of bed?				

	Always	Sometimes	Never	Don't Know
Can he or she normally walk without a cane, walker, or person?				
If not, does this person . . . walk alone using a walker?				
walk alone using a cane?				
walk only with someone assisting?				
normally use a wheelchair?				

Does this person . . .	Always	Sometimes	Never	Don't Know
have good balance when standing and walking?				
fall out of bed?				

Reprinted with permission from *The Alzheimer's Health Care Handbook: How to Get the Best Medical Care for Your Relative with Alzheimer's Disease, in and out of the Hospital,* by Mary S. Mittelman, DrPH and Cynthia Epstein, LCSW, 2002 Marlowe & Co, New York, Copyright 2002, 2003 by Mary S. Mittelman, DrPH.

Does this person . . .	Always	Sometimes	Never	Don't Know
lose personal possessions such as glasses etc.?				
get confused by new people?				
get confused in new places?				
get anxious or frightened if left alone?				
wander or pace?				
have angry outbursts or yell?				
get agitated or upset in the late afternoon?				
stay awake at night?				
become physically aggressive (biting, grabbing, spitting)?				
act in sexually inappropriate ways?				
have hallucinations, delusions or paranoia?				
often get depressed, sad or withdrawn?				

What helps calm this person when he or she becomes upset?	Always	Sometimes	Never	Don't Know
playing soothing music				
increasing the lights				
dimming the lights				
taking a walk				
offering food				
turning the television on				
turning the television off				
being with someone familiar				
being left alone				

Other things that help (*specify*)

_____

_____

_____

8. What medical conditions does this person have?

_____

_____

_____

_____

Reprinted with permission from *The Alzheimer's Health Care Handbook: How to Get the Best Medical Care for Your Relative with Alzheimer's Disease, in and out of the Hospital,* by Mary S. Mittelman, DrPH and Cynthia Epstein, LCSW, 2002 Marlowe & Co, New York, Copyright 2002, 2003 by Mary S. Mittelman, DrPH.

9. What medications does this person take?

(Be sure to include prescription and nonprescription drugs, vitamins, nutritional and herb supplements.)

Name of Medication	Dose	When Given	Name of Medication	Dose	When Given

10. Is this person allergic to any medicines?   *Yes   No   Don't Know*

If yes, which ones _____

_____

11. Is this person allergic to any foods?   *Yes   No   Don't Know*

If yes, which ones _____

_____

12. Does this person need a special diet or consistency of food?   *Yes   No   Don't Know*

If yes, please explain_____

_____

13. Is he or she enrolled in the Safe Return Program?   *Yes   No   Don't Know*

(If a Safe Return member gets lost, call 1-800-572-1122.)

14. Has the person with memory impairment completed advance directives?   *Yes   No   Don't Know*

If so, where can they be found?_____

15. Personal history of person with memory impairment

What kind of work does (or did) this person do? _____

_____

What are (or were) his or her interests or hobbies? _____

_____

Is there anything else that is important to know about this person, such as special needs or plans? _____

_____

Reprinted with permission from *The Alzheimer's Health Care Handbook: How to Get the Best Medical Care for Your Relative with Alzheimer's Disease, in and out of the Hospital,* by Mary S. Mittelman, DrPH and Cynthia Epstein, LCSW, 2002 Marlowe & Co, New York, Copyright 2002, 2003 by Mary S. Mittelman, DrPH.

Activities Schedule for Backup Caregiver (Sample Form)

Personal Needs	Yes	No	Where to Find
Cane	❐	❐	_____
Dentures	❐	❐	_____
Glasses	❐	❐	_____
Hearing aid	❐	❐	_____
Walker	❐	❐	_____

Morning Routine
Breakfast _____ Where Eaten _____
Amount of Help Needed _____
Special Utensils Needed _____
Medications with Meals ❐ _____ Nap ❐ _____
Snack Foods _____ Time of Snack _____

Evening Routine
Dinner _____ Where Eaten _____
Evening Snack _____

Bedtime Routine
Help Needed Undressing ❐ _____ Shower or Bath Needed ❐ _____
Where Clothes Are Stored _____
Where Dentures Are Stored _____
Special Items Needed: _____
Incontinent Pad/Brief ❐ _____ Urinal ❐ _____ Restraints ❐ _____
Special Pillows ❐ _____ Music ❐ _____ Nightlight ❐ _____
Calming Techniques _____
_____

Special Concerns or Equipment
Catheter ❐ _____ Oxygen ❐ _____
Special Precautions _____
Other _____
Resuscitate ❐   **Do Not Resuscitate** ❐

Be on the Alert for:
Gates on Stairs/Locks on Doors _____
Alarms _____
Other _____
Don't be surprised if: _____

Resources for Finding Paid Help

Use a Home Health Care Agency

Home Health Care Agencies are for-profit, nonprofit, or are run by the government. They provide personal care, skilled care, instructions for caregiver and care receiver, and supervision. They usually provide certified nurse assistants (CNAs), sometimes called home health aides; registered nurses (RNs); licensed practical nurses (LPNs); physical therapists, occupational therapists, and speech therapists. (A doctor's order is required in order to get coverage for skilled-care nursing in the home.) These agencies help plan services and care that match the health, social, and financial needs of the client.

Definitions for Agencies

There are a number of terms to describe an agency's services and how it is able to do what it does. Study the terms carefully before looking into the agencies in your area.

Accredited—Services have been reviewed by a nonprofit organization interested in quality home health care.

Bonded—The agency has paid a fixed dollar amount in order to be bonded. In the event of a court action the bond pays the penalties. (Being bonded does not ensure good service.)

Certified—The agency has met the minimum federal standards for care and takes part in the Medicare program.

Certified Health Personnel—Those who work for the agency meet the standards of a licensing agency for the state.

Insurance Claims Honored—The agency will look into insurance benefits and will accept assignment of benefits (meaning the insurance company pays the agency directly).

Licensed—The agency has met the requirements to run its business (in those states that oversee home health care agencies).

Licensed Health Personnel—The personnel (staff) of the agency have passed the state licensing exam for that profession.

Screened—References have been checked; a criminal background check may or may not have been made.

Types of Health Care Professionals

Registered Nurse (RN)—has at least 2 years of school training and is licensed by the state Board of Nursing Examiners

Licensed Practical Nurse (LPN)—has finished a one-year course of study and is licensed by the state Board of Licensed Vocational Nurses

Certified Nurses Aide (CNA)—has finished 70 hours of classes and 50 hours of clinical practice in a nursing center setting; must pass a test and register with the State Board of Nursing

Home Health Aide—is screened on the basis of work experience; training and requirements differ from state to state

Someone who is taking classes or is in a training program that leads to one of the above professions might be able to help with care.

Checklist **Things to Do Before Selecting an Agency**

✓ Interview several agencies.

✓ Get references and CHECK THEM.

✓ Make a list of services you want and ask the agency what it will cost.

✓ Ask what the steps are in the care planning and management process and how long each will take.

✓ Find out how and when you can contact the care manager.

✓ Find out if the agency has a system for sending a substitute (stand-in) aide if the regular one doesn't show up.

✓ Ask if the agency will replace the aide if that aide and the person in care do not get along.

✓ Ask about the skills and ongoing training of personnel.

✓ Do they have staff especially trained to work with dementia?

✓ Ask how they keep track of the quality of services.

✓ Ask for the services needed by the person in care, even if the insurance company is trying to hold down costs.

✓ Be aware that if a social service agency is providing the care services, they may limit you to only the services that they provide.

✓ Ask them to tell you about any referral-fee agreements they may have with nursing homes or other care facilities.

✓ Know what you have to do to lodge complaints against the agency with the state ombudsman or long-term-care office.

✓ Get in touch with the local/state Division for Aging Services to check for complaints against a particular agency.

How to Screen a Personal Hire

- Check licenses, training, experience, and references.
- Run a criminal background check and a driving record check (through a private investigator). Also, ask to see the person's insurance card.
- Find out if the person has a special skill (for example, working with care receivers who have dementia).
- Decide whether the person is someone who can meet the emotional needs of the person in your care.
- Consider his or her personal habits.
- Find out if he is a smoker or nonsmoker.

 NOTE You can hire a private investigator to look at public records and check on education and licenses, driving history, and previous employers. This service can be obtained anywhere in the country.

Questions to Ask of the Applicant's References:

When someone is going to be hired, ask for the names of people who can tell you about this person's work and personal habits. Here are some questions you can ask:

- How long have you known this person?
- Did this person work for you?
- Is this person reliable, on time for work, patient, able to adjust as things change, able to be trusted, and polite?
- How does this person handle disagreements and emergencies?
- How well does this person follow directions, respond to requests, and take advice?

Paying for Care

You can look to many sources for help in paying for care. Some are public, while others are private or volunteer. The most common ways to pay for home care are as follows:

- personal and family resources
- private insurance
- Medicare, Medicaid, Department of Veterans Affairs, and Title programs
- community-based services

Because Alzheimer's disease is a progressive disease the type of care needed changes with time. You must consider the costs you face today as well as those you will face later on, as the dementia gets worse.

Assessment of Financial Resources

First, complete a personal financial resources assessment by doing the following steps:

- Look at current assets, where the care receiver's income comes from, and insurance entitlements.
- Prepare a budget and figure out what his future income might be from all sources.
- Confirm the qualifications, retirement benefits, and Social Security status of the person in your care.
- Figure as closely as possible the expenses of professional care and equipment. Include any medical procedures for other conditions likely to be needed.
- Check on the person's personal tax status and find out what care items and expenses are deductible.
- Find out if the person's health insurance or employer's workers' compensation policy has home health care benefits.

- Figure out how much money the person will need.
- If the person with AD doesn't have enough money to pay for care you may need to consider whether you can provide financial help.

 NOTE Think about making the person in your care a "dependent" and thus be able to transfer medical expenses to a taxpayer who can make use of medical deductions.

The cost of long-term care for a person with dementia can be very expensive. People often assume that government programs pay for care. In fact, individuals and families usually pay for care themselves. Advance planning can ease this burden.

Public Pay Programs

Medicare

Medicare is a federal health insurance program. It provides health care benefits to all Americans 65 and older and to those who have been determined to be "disabled" according to the Social Security Administration. There are constant changes in Medicare policies, requirements, and forms. Therefore, it is always best to get the most current information on benefits by calling the Medicare Hotline (📖 p. 82) or your hospital's social worker.

Things That Affect Medicare Eligibility

Whether the Person Is Homebound—Medicare will pay for certain home health care services only if the person is confined to the home and requires part-time skilled (nursing) services or therapy. Medicare does not cover ongoing custodial (maintenance) care. "Confined to home" does not mean bedridden. It means that a person cannot leave home except for medical care and requires help to get there. (Brief absences from the home do not affect eligibility.)

In order for treatments, services, and supplies to be paid for, they must be ordered by a doctor. They must also be provided by a home health agency certified by Medicare and the state health department.

Whether Care Is Intermittent (periodic)—In order to be covered, skilled services are required. Medicare is not designed to meet chronic ongoing needs that are considered "custodial" rather than "skilled."

Medicare Generally Pays for the Following:

- almost all costs of skilled care, such as doctors, nurses, and specialists
- various types of therapy—occupational, physical, speech-language
- home health services
- medical supplies and equipment
- personal care by home health aides (such as bathing, dressing, fixing meals, even light housekeeping and counseling) after discharge from a hospital or nursing home

NOTE Phrases like "intermittent care," "skilled care," and "homebound" are not precisely defined. They are different from region to region, and the type and availability of coverage by Medicare may be different as well.

Services NOT covered by Medicare

Full-time nursing care at home, meals delivered to the home, homemaker chore services *not* related to care, and personal care services are usually not covered by Medicare.

A caregiver who has power of attorney for a person on Medicare (the beneficiary) must send written evidence to the person's Medicare Part B carrier. Send a letter with the person's name, number, signature, and a statement that the caregiver can act on behalf of the beneficiary. The form must list start and end dates.

If there is a dispute about a repayment from Medicare, a review may be requested by filing a claim with the Medicare carrier.

Medicare Part B Insurance

Medicare Part B insurance offers extra benefits to basic Medicare coverage. It pays for tests, doctor's office visits, lab services, and home health care.

Medicare Supplemental Insurance (Medigap)

To pay for benefits not covered by Medicare, this private health insurance option is available. It pays for noncovered services only—for example, hospital deductibles, doctor copayments, and eyeglasses—but does not cover long-term care services. Coverage depends on the plan you buy.

For anyone who has Medicare HMO coverage, Medigap insurance may not be necessary because those individuals only make a small copayment but do not pay a deductible for doctor's visits.

NOTE It is illegal for an insurance company or agent to sell you a second Medigap policy unless you put in writing that you intend to end the Medigap policy you have. The federal toll-free telephone number for filing complaints is (800) 633-4227.

Medicaid pays for the medical care of low-income elderly persons or those whose assets have been used up while paying for their own care. Eligibility depends on monthly income limits and personal assets. Coverage includes nursing facilities, assisted living, foster care, and certain types of home care. Each state runs its own Medicaid program, and so eligibility and coverage can vary. Some states have set up Medicaid Waiver programs, which pay for home and community-based services that would otherwise only be paid if one were in a nursing home.

Common Aspects of Medicaid

- Recipients must be financially and medically in need.

- For recipients who are terminally ill, benefits go on for as long as they are ill. However, care must be provided by an agency with hospice certification and Medicaid certification.

- Payments are made directly to providers of services.

- Long-term-care costs are paid for those not covered by insurance and for patients whose finances have run out.

- Payments to foster care homes and retirement communities are not covered (except in some cases by Medicaid waiver).

- Home health care services, medical supplies, and equipment are covered.

- Eligibility is based on a person's income and assets.

- People with disabilities who are eligible for state public assistance are eligible for Medicaid.

- People with disabilities eligible for Supplemental Social Security (SSI) are eligible for Medicaid.

- In many states, there are laws (called spousal impoverishment laws) that protect a portion of the estate and assets for the healthy spouse. These come into play after other monies have been "spent down" for the care of the ill spouse.

To find out what the benefits are, contact the local Social Security office, city or county public assistance office, or the Area Agency on Aging.

Services NOT covered by Medicaid

As a rule, Medicare, Medicaid, and private insurance do not cover many in-home services because they are not medical services. However, some community services may be called on to fill the gap for free or on a subsidized (public funding) basis. The following services usually are not covered but might be available locally free of charge:

- social model adult day care
- alcohol and drug programs
- case management
- household chore services
- neighborhood and local meal services, such as Meals on Wheels
- consumer protection
- emergency response systems (which provide contact by phone or electronic device to police and rescue services)
- emergency assistance for food, clothing, or shelter
- friendly visitors (volunteers who stop by to write letters or run errands)
- services and equipment for those who have disabilities
- homemaker services
- legal and financial services
- respite care

- senior centers

- support groups

- telephone reassurance (volunteers who make calls to or receive calls from those who are elderly or living alone)

A note on adult day care: Adult day care follows two models—a *medical* model and a *social* model. Medical models offer medical supervision and hands-on care to frail elderly and people with dementia and may be covered by Medicaid. The social model provides respite care, supervision, personal care, and social stimulation, but is generally not paid for by Medicaid.

NOTE The U.S. Congress continually makes changes to Medicare and Medicaid, which will affect payment for acute and long-term care. As these changes are put into effect, they are posted on the Web site of the Center for Medicare and Medicaid Services (CMS): www.cms.gov

NOTE After symptoms of Alzheimer's appear, one usually cannot buy most kinds of insurance.

NOTE Life insurance can be a source of cash. The person with AD may be able to receive part of the face value of the policy as a loan called a critical loan, that is paid off when the person dies.

Consumer-Directed Model of Care

In some states, under a special waiver program called Consumer-Directed Care, Medicaid beneficiaries do not have to use a designated Medicaid agency but can select their own provider. Depending on the particular state guidelines, the person may be a family member or other suitable person who will be paid by Medicaid for providing a certain number of hours of care to be determined by the program.

The benefit of this program is that it allows the family to select a provider. However, they may also be responsible for providing a back-up person should the primary provider not be available. You should review the conditions of this program in your state and decide whether it meets your needs.

Department of Veterans Affairs Benefits

Veterans generally qualify for health services in the home if a disability is service related. Even if a disability is not service related, other benefits may be available based on income qualifications. Some states have special programs only for veterans who live in that state. Some Veterans Hospitals have programs to deliver home health care services. Contact the nearest Veterans Affairs office or veterans group in your area.

Older Americans Act and Social Services Block Grant

Some agencies that provide support services get funding under this program. Services available may include the following:

- case management and assessment
- household chore services (minor household repairs, cleaning, yard work)
- companion services

- community meals
- home-delivered hot meals (Meals on Wheels) once or twice a day
- homemaker services
- transportation

Long-Term-Care Insurance

If the person in your care has long-term-care insurance, review the policy's criteria for hiring help. You may want to consider purchasing long-term-care insurance for *yourself* so that *your* future care needs are covered.

In view of the number of years a person may live with AD, it is possible that long-term-care benefits may end while the person still requires ongoing care. It is necessary to consider that this may happen when planning for the financial future of the person with AD, his spouse, or other family members.

Private Pay

After you have reviewed all the ways in which care can be paid for, you may find that you have to or want to pay for care yourself. If there is a possibility that other family members may be willing to contribute to the cost, discuss it with them and perhaps together you can make a plan that everyone accepts to reduce the financial burden on one person.

Tip Choose a financial adviser who is familiar with elder care.

Many states license individuals to offer analysis of insurance coverage for a fee. In some states if a person has a license to sell and a license to counsel, he or she can only perform one of those services for a specific client. Check your state department of insurance for information about insurance counselors.

 Consult a professional before making decisions.

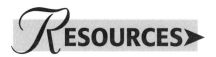 **ESOURCES**▶

AARP
601 E. Street, NW
Washington, D.C. 20049
(800) 424-3410
www.aarp.org
Provides information on Medicare benefits.

Alzheimer's Association
225 N. Michigan Ave.
Fl. 17
Chicago, IL 60601
24-hour Helpline (800) 272-3900
www.alz.org
The Alzheimer's Association CareFinder
www.alz.org/carefinder/index.asp
Provides support and information for AD patients and their families.

CareScout
(800) 571-1918
www.carescout.com
Care advocates help thousands of families each year find the most appropriate home health aides, homemakers, assisted living facilities, and nursing homes.

The Center for Applied Gerontology, Council for Jewish Elderly
3003 W. Touhy Avenue
Chicago, IL 60645.
(773) 508-1000
E-mail: cag@cje.net
www.cje.net/professional/cag_orderform_2.pdf
Offers a 32-page pamphlet "Someone Who Cares: A Guide to Hiring an In-Home Caregiver." *$9.95 plus $3.50 shipping and handling.*

Centers for Medicare and Medicaid Services
7500 Security Boulevard
Baltimore, MD 21244-1850
(800) MEDICARE (633-4227) Medicare Hotline
www.cms.gov
www.medicare.gov
Federal agency that administers the Medicare and Medicaid programs, including hospice benefits.

Eldercare Locator
(800) 677-1116
www.eldercare.gov
The local AAA is one of the first resources a family caregiver for an adult 60 years or older should contact when help is needed. Almost every state has one or more AAA, which serves local communities, older residents, and their families. Local AAAs are generally listed in the city or county government sections of the telephone directory under "Aging" or "Social Services." A caregiver can identify the nearest AAA by contacting the Eldercare Locator.

Family Caregiver Alliance
690 Market Street, Suite 600
San Francisco, CA 94104
(800) 445-8106; 415-434-3388 Fax: (415) 434-3508
www.caregiver.org
E-mail: info@caregiver.org
Resource center for caregivers of people with chronic disabling conditions. The Web site provides information on services and programs in education, research, and advocacy.

National Association for Home Care
228 Seventh Street, SE
Washington, DC 20003
(202) 547-7424
www.nahc.org
Provides referrals to state associations, which can refer callers to local agencies. Offers publications, including the free pamphlet "How to Choose a Home Care Agency: A Consumer's Guide." Information on finding help, interviewing, reference checking, training, being a good manager, maintaining a good working and personal relationship, problems that might arise and how best to solve them, service dogs, assistive technology, and tax responsibilities. Contains sample forms and letters.

National Association of Area Agencies on Aging
(800) 677-1116
www.eldercare.gov
www.aoa.dhhs.gov
Supplies information about many eldercare issues, including respite care. Provides referrals to local respite programs and local Area Agency on Aging.

National Association of Professional Geriatric Care Managers
1604 N. Country Club Road
Tucson, AZ 85716
(520) 881-8008
www.caremanager.org
Their Web site provides a free list of care managers in your state.

The National Council on the Aging
300 D Street SW, Suite 801
Washington, D.C. 20024
(202) 479-1200
www.ncoa.org
Provides a link to benefits (www.benefitscheckup.org) that helps seniors find state and federal benefits programs.

National Family Caregivers Association
10400 Connecticut Avenue, Suite 500
Kensington, MD 20895-3944
(800) 896-3650; (301) 942-6430
www.thefamilycaregiver.org
Email: info@thefamilycaregiver.org
The Association supports, empowers, educates, and speaks up for more than 50 million Americans who care for a chronically ill, aged, or disabled person.

Publications

Avoiding Attendants from Hell: A Practical Guide to Finding, Hiring and Keeping Personal Care Attendants by June Price, Science and Humanities Press

Managing Personal Assistants: A Consumer Guide, published by Paralyzed Veterans of America. To purchase a copy call (888) 860-7244, or download online at www.pva.org/cgi-bin/pvastore/products.cgi?id=2

If you don't have access to the Internet, ask your local library to help you locate a Web site.

Financial, Legal, and Medical Planning

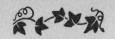

Financial, Legal, and Medical Planning

*I*t is important to decide how future health care, legal, and financial decisions will be made **before** things reach the crisis stage and the person with dementia can't participate. These decisions should be recorded in legal documents for two reasons:

- *to make sure that a person's wishes are honored*
- *to make sure the family has enough information about those wishes in order to make life-and-death decisions*

The ability to plan for future decisions depends on one's ability to:

- *understand the available choices*
- *understand the results of those options*
- *make and communicate a thoughtful choice*
- *express values and goals*

Once these matters are understood, a range of legal documents can be drawn up to help ensure that the person's wishes will be carried out.

The following information is not intended as legal advice. We have presented a general summary of the rights of capable adults to make, or arrange for others to make, their health care decisions. Our summary does not contain all the technical details of laws in each state. Check what your state requires by law.

Financial and Legal Planning for People with Alzheimer's

There are many legal tools that can help you and the person in your care now and in the future. Financial and legal planning is necessary and should be started early. Planning for the future should include looking at income tax issues, protecting existing assets, saving for the future, and paying for care. Long-term planning will help you and the person with AD feel more secure, no matter what the future brings.

You should also seek advice about insurance, employment rights, and state- assistance programs. If possible, discuss all options with the person in your care.

Caregivers need to understand the Social Security benefits and insurance policies of the person in their care, including medical insurance, Medicare, and private disability insurance. Familiarize yourself with the covered expenses, copayments and deductibles. Caregivers also need to understand the Americans with Disabilities Act (ADA) and other laws that are designed to protect housing, transportation, recreation, and employment.

When planning for the future, expert advice can be helpful, as the laws change and depend on where you live. It may feel overwhelming to have to make all these arrangements. Many community agencies offer legal and financial planning services. Contact your local chapter of the Alzheimer's Association for information and resources.

NOTE Financial planning will assure that your property—no matter how little you have—goes to the people you choose as quickly and as cheaply as possible.

Financial and Legal Planning Tools

Will—a legal document that spells out how money and property is to be given out after death. If a person is disabled or does not have the physical or mental abilities to tend to his or her own affairs, other legal papers are needed.

Living Trust—a legal document that names someone (a trustee) to manage a person's finances or assets. A trust includes advice on how to manage assets and when to distribute them (give them out). It can also protect assets from probate, which is a long legal process to make sure that the will is legal. Usually, the trust goes into effect if a person becomes unable to function well and is likely to make bad financial decisions.

Power of Attorney—a document that names someone to make decisions about money and property for a person who is unable to make those decisions. A person should have one power of attorney for financial management and a separate power of attorney for health care.

Representative Payee—someone named by the Social Security Administration to manage a person's Social Security benefits when that person is unable to look after his or her own money and bill paying.

Conservatorship—a legal proceeding in which the court names an individual to handle another's finances when that person becomes unable to do so.

Making a will, setting up a trust, providing income, and protecting assets may involve future decisions about giving to charity, insurance policies, annuities (yearly payments), and other instruments. This kind of planning is necessary and should not be put off.

NOTE ▶ If the person in your care is in the early stage of AD, and still able to make plans for the future, it is a good idea to suggest he prepare a letter of instructions. The letter should list all property and debts, location of the original will and other important documents, and names and addresses of professional advisors. It should also include funeral wishes and special instructions for giving away personal property such as furniture and jewelry.

Guardianship

If the person in your care did not choose someone to act on his behalf when he was still competent, preparing Advance Directives such as a General Durable Power of Attorney and Healthcare Power of Attorney, it may be necessary for you to formally become his guardian so you can make decisions on his behalf.

A legal action seeking appointment of a guardian will avoid conflict with others who may not agree with your decisions and empower you to act for the person in your care. This will involve a court procedure for which you will need legal representation. A court must find a person to be mentally incapacitated and in need of someone to step in as decision-maker before a guardian will be appointed on his or her behalf.

The responsibilities of a guardian may include deciding where the person lives, the personal and medical care he or she receives, and how his financial resources are used.

STORING DOCUMENTS

Store—Death certificates, military records, tax returns for the last six years, pension documents

Keep in the safe-deposit box—Original will, deeds, passport, stock and bond certificates, birth and marriage certificates, insurance policies

Keep at home—a copy of the will that is in the safe deposit box

Throw out—expired insurance policies, checks that are more than one year old and are not tax-related

Health Care Decision Making and Alzheimer's Disease

It is important to remember that in the early stage of Alzheimer's disease, the person with dementia may still be physically strong and may also have serious memory problems, but it is likely that he can still make his preferences about treatment known. His choices should be followed whenever possible. Because of the progressive nature of the disease, it is especially important that advance directives be considered while the person with dementia can be involved in making decisions for himself. Once the severe stage is reached it may become necessary to decide whether to continue treating or curing any illness that the person with dementia has or whether to begin palliative (treating pain without trying to cure) care. Without an advance directive, life-prolonging measures may still be performed, even though hope of recovery is gone.

If there is disagreement among family members and there is no advance directive, it may be necessary for the court to appoint a guardian to be decision maker.

 It is easier to think about having an autopsy in advance; if one is desired, it should be part of the advance directives.

Directives for Health Care

There are two types of legal documents for indicating a person's wishes for advance directives if he or she is not able to make his or her own decisions. One type outlines the kind of medical attention the person wants, and the other names the person who will make sure these wishes are carried out. (The names of the documents may be different in your state.)

Discussing the Person's Wishes

- When possible, discuss the person's and the family's wishes before an illness reaches the final phase.
- Does the person have a Health Care Proxy?
- Is there a living will or medical power of attorney?
- What would the person's choices be regarding life support?
- Would the person want to stay at home or enter a facility?

Living Will

A living will spells out a person's wishes about medical care in case he or she is physically unable to state those wishes. When drawing up a living will, it is important to consider a person's attitudes and desires regarding health care. (📖 See p. 244, for having one's wishes honored while traveling.)

Health Care Proxy (Health Care Power of Attorney or Advance Directive)

This document allows a person to name someone as a personal representative (the health care proxy or representative) and gives that person the authority, or right, to carry out the person's wishes, as outlined in the living will.

Do Not Resuscitate Order (DNR)

This document instructs medical personnel not to use CPR (cardiopulmonary resuscitation) if the person's heart stops beating.

Values History

This document explains a person's views on life and death and what he or she thinks is important. This can help the proxy or representative understand the person's wishes. It is a very helpful document because there is no way of knowing every medical situation that can possibly happen.

Why It Makes Sense to Prepare Directives

- They can be flexible and tailored to an individual's wishes.

- They apply to all health care situations.

- They may be given to anyone—a friend, relative, or spiritual advisor—to hold until needed.

- They are honored in the state where they were written and in most other states (check the state in question).

- They are not limited to issues of prolonging life but can also, for example, cover dental work and surgery.

- They can be created by filling out a standard form.

- Advance Health Care Directive forms are different from state to state and are available from most hospitals and nursing homes.

- They can be revoked (cancelled) at any time as long as the person is mentally able.

It is important to have these legal and health documents for the person you are caring for. It is also important that you, the caregiver, have these documents drawn up for yourself.

If, in the past, you designated the person who is now in your care as *your* decision maker, then someone else must be selected. It can feel very sad to realize that the person you counted on to protect you will not be able to do so. It is nevertheless essential that you find an alternative person.

Health Maintenance Organizations (HMOs)

Health Maintenance Organizations are prepaid health insurance plans that give complete medical coverage for a fixed premium. Knowing whether an HMO is right for

Checklist Do's and Don'ts in Planning Health Care

✓ Do execute a new power of attorney or directive every few years to show that your wishes have not changed.

✓ Do use the proper form for your state.

✓ Do have the document drawn up by a lawyer so it follows the state rules.

✓ Do give a copy to the doctor, hospital, and any person holding power of attorney.

✓ Do ask the doctor and lawyer of the person in your care to review the document while that person is competent (mentally and physically able). Make sure they accept what is in it.

✓ Do keep a card with health care information in your wallet or that of the person in your care.

✓ Don't name the doctor as power of attorney.

✓ Do carry a copy of the document with you when you travel. (📖 See **Travel**, p. 244.)

the person in your care requires careful study. Before enrolling the person in your care in an HMO it is essential that you verify that she will have access to specialists in dementia care and any other illness the person may have.

Planning Funeral Arrangements

To ensure that the wishes of a dying person are carried out and to decrease the level of stress on the family at the time of death, it is helpful for the family to discuss all aspects of the death and all funeral arrangements while the person is still alive and can participate in the discussion. Planning in advance will ensure that the person's wishes are carried out with a minimum of cost. The simpler the service the less expensive it will be, but remember that ritual is important to a bereaved family. Contact funeral homes in your area for specific details.

If your area has a nonprofit memorial association, its volunteers have likely done price comparisons of local funeral homes.

NOTE People often place their funeral instructions in a safe-deposit box that may not be opened until after the funeral. It is better to keep the instructions where they can be easily located and to give a copy to the nearest relative.

Information That Will Be Needed After Death

Many facts can be gathered in a person's lifetime and recorded in a simple Estate Planner. Keep this little booklet or form (available from most funeral homes, some attorneys, and stationery stores) in a safe place and let the family know where it is located.

Be sure you have telephone numbers for the following people so you can reach them easily:

- accountant
- attorney
- business associates
- clergy
- doctor
- employees
- employer
- estate executor or trustee
- family
- financial advisor

- friends
- funeral home where the funeral is pre-planned
- health representative, if other than you
- tax preparer

Financial Information to Record in Your Estate Planner

In an estate planning booklet or informal list, keep clear records of the following information, complete with account numbers, addresses, telephone numbers, and the location of the documents:

- investments, their amounts, and brokers
- annuities
- bank checking and savings accounts
- life insurance with policy numbers
- Medicare and supplemental insurance
- military service and veterans' benefits
- mortgages and liabilities
- pension plans, profit-sharing, Keogh plans, and IRAs
- real estate holdings
- safe-deposit box location and key
- Social Security card and number and the date benefits began, if applicable
- workers compensation, if applicable
- list of motor vehicles owned and location of titles

Survivors' Benefits

Carefully check all life and casualty insurance and death benefits. Check on income for survivors from a credit union, trade union, fraternal organization, the military, and the Social Security Administration. Some debts and installment payments may carry insurance clauses that will cancel them. Consult with creditors if there will be a delay in payments and ask for more time.

Social Security Benefits

The widow, dependent widower, children, and dependent parents of an insured person may be eligible for monthly survivors' payments. (They usually don't start for about six weeks). However, Social Security benefits are not paid automatically. To apply, you will need the following documents:

- birth certificate of the deceased
- marriage certificate
- birth certificates of survivors (under 22 years of age if they are full-time college students; under 18 if they are not)
- proof of widow's or widower's age, if 62 or older
- proof of termination of any preceding marriage
- record of income for the preceding year

The surviving spouse or minor children may also receive a modest one-time death benefit. Ask your Social Security office for help in filling out your claims.

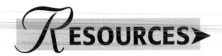

AARP
(800) 424-3410
www.aarp.com
E-mail: griefandloss@aarp.org
Offers a grief and loss counseling program run by volunteers who have experienced loss.

AARP Tax-Aide
www.aarp.org/taxaide/home.htm (for a listing of site locations)
(888) 227-7669
Call 24 hours a day, 7 days a week to find a site near you. Provides free help on federal, state and local tax returns to middle- and low-income persons aged 60 years and older; also provides online counselors at the Web site. This program also accepts volunteers.

Administration on Aging
www.aoa.gov/legal/hotline.html
Web site lists legal hotlines for the states that have them for those 60 and older.

Caring Connections
(800) 658-8898
www.caringinfo.org
Distributes state-specific forms and explanatory guides for creating a living will.

Certified Financial Planners Board of Standards
(800) 487-1497; (303) 830-7500; (888) 237-6275
www.cfp-board.org
This organization will provide information on whether a planner is certified, how long he or she has been certified, and if any disciplinary action has ever been taken.

Deceased Do Not Contact List
www.preference.the-dma.org/cgi/ddnc.php
Removes deceased people's names from mailing lists.

The Equal Justice Network
www.equaljustice.org/hotline
A Web site sponsored by programs in the field offering legal advice over the telephone.

Financial Planning Association
Suite 400, 4100 E. Mississippi Ave.
Denver, CO 80246-3053
(800) 322-4237 Fax (404) 845-3660
www.fpanet.org
Web site provides a list and backgrounds of certified financial planners in your region and a helpful free pamphlet, Selecting a Qualified Financial Planning Professional, which lists questions you should ask a financial planner before hiring him or her.

Funeral Consumers Alliance
33 Patchen Road
South Burlington, VT 05403
(800) 765-0107
www.funerals.org
Provides information about alternatives for funeral or non-funeral dispositions; can refer you to individual Societies in the state of your choice.

Funeral Service Consumer Assistance Program
P.O. Box 486
Elm Grove, WI 53122-0486
(800) 662-7666
www.fsef.org
Provides help to consumers and funeral directors to resolve disagreements about funeral service contracts; provides referrals and information on death, grief and funeral service.

Gift of Hope Organ & Tissue Donor Network
(888) 307-3668
www.giftofhope.org

IRS Web Site
(800) 829-3676 for publications; (800) 829-1040 for answers to tax questions
www.irs.gov
The Web site provides tax forms. Form 559 is for survivors, and Form 524 is for those who are elderly or disabled.

Last Acts
www.lastacts.org
Comprehensive Web site with links to resources for end-of-life care.

National Academy of Elder Law Attorneys
1604 N. Country Club Road
Tucson, AZ 85716
(520) 881-4005
www.naela.org
Provides a list of member lawyers in your area.

National Association of Personal Financial Advisors
www.napfa.org

Older Women's League
3300 N. Fairfax Drive, Suite 218
Arlington, VA 22201
(800) 825-3695; (703) 812-7990
Fax (703) 812-0687
www.owl-national.org

Public Reference Branch
Federal Trade Commission
Sixth Street & Pennsylvania Avenue, N.W.
Washington, D. C. 20580
For the free brochure "Facts for Consumers: Funerals A Consumer Guide," send a self-addressed, stamped envelope.

Social Security Administration
(800) 772-1213
www.socialsecurity.gov
Provides a personal report on a person's Social Security record.

Society of Financial Service Professionals
www.financialpro.org

Call your local **Social Security Administration, State Health Department, State Hospice Organization**, or call (800) 633-4227 **Medicare Hotline** to learn about hospice benefits.

If you don't have home access to the Internet, ask your local library to help you locate any Web site.

Laughter is the best medicine.

Gentlemen, why don't you laugh? With the fearful strain that is upon me day and night, if I did not laugh I should die, and you need this medicine as much as I do.

— Abraham Lincoln during the Civil War

Health Care for the Person with Alzheimer's Disease

Health Care for the Person with Alzheimer's Disease

*A*lzheimer's disease may not make people feel physically ill, but AD does get in the way of them keeping themselves healthy. That is why they must rely on their caregivers to help them to eat a balanced diet, take their medications correctly, visit the doctor, and take care of all the details that are involved in staying in good physical and emotional health. Even at the very beginning of the illness, a person with Alzheimer's disease will need help to manage the self-care that is needed to stay as fit as his age allows.

Routine Health Care

People with Alzheimer's disease are generally elderly, so it is not surprising that they may need glasses, hearing aids, or dentures, just like other older adults. It is important to be sure that all of these aids that help a person to interact with other people, and to enjoy the simple pleasures of eating, reading, and taking part in social activities are in good condition and are checked regularly. When a person with AD does not see or hear well, she may be even more confused and be left out of activities she still might be able to enjoy. In addition to Alzheimer's disease, the person may also have other illnesses such as high blood pressure, diabetes, and cancer, which also need to be treated.

> **NOTE** It is important to have a doctor who is willing to work with other health care providers, understands Alzheimer's disease, is respectful of the person in your care, and is prepared to include *you*, in the decision-making process. The doctor should also be concerned about how *you*, the caregiver, are holding up under the stress.

These are some of the routine medical interventions you will want the person to have—

- regular annual complete check ups
- flu and pneumonia vaccinations
- screening for other medical conditions, as recommended by the doctor

It may be useful for the person to be seen by a geriatric pyschiatrist in addition to medical doctors to get a complete picture of his physical and emotional health.

Even if the person with Alzheimer's disease seems to be feeling well, it is important for the doctor to examine him. A condition the person with dementia was unable to tell you about may be found and treated before it becomes more serious.

Sometimes a condition you did not know about before may be discovered by the doctor, and you will have to choose among different ways of treating it or decide if you want to treat it at all. You always need to keep in mind that a person with Alzheimer's disease may have difficulty cooperating with certain treatments because he may not understand why they are necessary. If the person is in the early stage, see if the treatment plan can be explained in a way the person will understand so that he can voice his opinions. Even if the person forgets what he said he would like or not like to have done, at least you will know. Ideally, you and the person in your care will have already completed the health care documents, called Advance Directives and Health Care Proxy (see *Financial, Legal, and Medical Planning,* p. 85), so that you will know how the person would like to be medically treated.

Take care of medical procedures such as cataract surgery as soon as they are recommended by the doctor. This way she will get the benefit sooner. In addition, in the earlier stage of dementia, she will be more likely to be able to handle the stress of the surgery and cooperate with the aftercare.

What will you need to do to be sure the person's health is properly cared for? That depends on the stage of the illness.

NOTE It is very important to have a written health history of the person with AD so there is a permanent record that health care providers can read when the person can no longer give his history for himself. (See Profile of a Patient with Memory Impairment, pp. 62–66.)

Early-Stage Routine Health Care

In the early stage of dementia (see *Understanding Alzheimer's Disease,* p. 3) you will—

- need to remind a person to take his medication
- check to see that he is taking the right medication at the right time
- reorder medications when necessary
- make appointments with doctors for him
- accompany the person with AD to the doctor
- bring lists of medications he is taking

- be prepared to give a medical health history if the doctor does not already know the person

- describe his symptoms

Middle-Stage Routine Health Care

When the person with AD advances to the middle stage of dementia, you will have more to do. He may be less *able* to cooperate with you, may refuse to take necessary medications or eat regularly or do other activities necessary to stay healthy. These behaviors sometimes are called *resistance to care.* They are the challenging behaviors for which medications are often recommended so the person may be less upset, angry, or difficult for the caregiver to manage. However, these medications can have serious side effects and are usually not as helpful as expected (see *Understanding Behavior in Alzheimer's Disease,* p. 200).

Some of the symptoms at this stage, such as hallucinations, delusions, and paranoia, are similar to those of people who have a mental illness. Although AD is *not* a mental illness, some of the same medications are prescribed. As mentioned above, while these drugs may be helpful, like all drugs, they must be used with caution, in the lowest possible doses, and checked often to see if they are working. Ask the doctor what side effects to look out for. If problems occur, ask if the person should switch to another medication or stop taking them.

NOTE If the behavior of a person with Alzheimer's disease changes suddenly or if a symptom appears that usually occurs much later in the illness **THINK MEDICAL ILLNESS** and call the doctor. Alzheimer's disease progresses slowly and any sudden change in behavior probably happened because the person is sick.

Common causes of these sudden behavior changes are:

- infection, such as a urinary tract infection
- dehydration
- constipation or diarrhea
- a broken bone

Late-Stage Routine Health Care

In the late stage of Alzheimer's disease, you will have to speak for the person with dementia and tell medical providers what type of care the person had said he wanted when he could still communicate his wishes.

 NOTE Note: Even when a person is in the early stage of AD, he may be in the late stage of *another* illness. The effects of *both* conditions on the person's decision-making ability and the likely outcome of a medical procedure should be taken into account when making decisions about the kind of care needed or whether it should be provided.

Remember: A person with Alzheimer's disease may not be able to tell you he is sick but may *show* you instead. Increased confusion, listlessness, change in walking, being less attentive, and loss of interest in eating may signal a physical illness.

Recording and Managing Medications

Always be sure that the person in your care takes the medication exactly as prescribed. Keep an accurate list of these medications and when they should be taken.

Never make any changes to these medications without talking to the doctor or specialist first. However, because everyone's treatment needs are different, the specialist may want to try changing the amount or timing of drugs, within certain limits. If you are worried or have any questions, don't be afraid to ask your doctor or pharmacist for advice.

People who have serious health problems often take a large number of medications at many different times of the day. It is essential to have a careful system for keeping track of medications:

- when medications should be given

- how they should be given

- when they were actually given

The following sample of a weekly medication schedule is a good model to follow. Be sure to fill in the times when (A.M. and P.M.) medications actually were given, and have each caregiver initial them.

As you prepare your own schedule, be sure to record information from the label of each prescription, including

- days of the week when each medicine must be taken

- number of times per day

- time of day

- whether the medicine is to be taken with or without food

- how much water should be taken with the medicine

Also make a note to yourself about any warnings (for example, "Don't take this medicine with alcohol") and possible side effects (dizziness, confusion, headache, etc.).

Weekly Medication Schedule (Sample Form)

Medication	Date/Time/Initials						
Name, dose, frequency, with or without food	Sat.	Sun.	Mon.	Tues.	Wed.	Thurs.	Fri.
Example							
Coumadin 2mg 1x daily a.m. with food							
Folic acid 400mg 1x daily a.m.							
Vitamin/mineral capsule 1x daily, with food • Noon							
Artificial tears 2x daily • 8 a.m. • bedtime							

NOTE Labels may contain the following abbreviations that you should be aware of:

HS—hour of sleep (medication time)
BID—give the medicine 2 times per day (approximately 8am and 8pm)
TID—give the medicine 3 times per day (approximately 9am, 1pm, 6pm)
QID—give the medicine 4 times per day (approximately 9am, 1pm, 5pm, 9pm)

Other Cautions

- Never crush drugs without talking to the doctor or pharmacist first. If the person in your care has trouble swallowing medication, ask the doctor if there is another way it can be taken.

- If the person in your care will take the medicine without your help, ask the pharmacist to use easy-open caps on prescription bottles.

- Do not store medicine that will be taken internally (swallowed) in the same cabinet with medicine that will be used externally (lotions, salves, creams, etc.)

- Keep a magnifying glass near the medicine cabinet for reading small print.

- Store most medicine in a cool, dry place—usually not the bathroom.

- Remove the cotton from each bottle so that moisture is not drawn in.

- Check with your pharmacist about disposal options for expired medications in your area.

- If childproof containers are too hard to open, ask the pharmacist for containers that are not childproof and be sure they are not available to the person with AD.

Tips for Getting the Person with AD to Take Medication

- Put the pills in a box that has sections for time of day and day of the week.

- Put the pills next to the person's plate at mealtime.

- Tell her she can have a treat after taking the medicine.

- Ask the pharmacist if it is okay to crush the pills and put them in food.

- If the person in your care has trouble swallowing pills, ask the doctor to prescribe liquid medicine or a patch.

- If the person refuses to take the medicine, wait a few minutes and ask again.

- Tell her the doctor called to ask if the medication was taken and you need to call back with an answer.

- Ask someone else to offer the medicine, the person may respond differently to him or her.

- Calmly offer the medicine while she is busy doing something else.

EMERGENCY PREPAREDNESS

Let the local fire station and ambulance company know that a person with disabilities lives at your address. They will have the information on hand and can respond quickly.

Visiting the Doctor

Here are some suggestions to make getting to the doctor easier:

- Leave plenty of time to get to the appointment. You cannot hurry a person with Alzheimer's. Any pressure to hurry up usually results only in upset. Just try to keep the focus on getting ready to leave.

- Get yourself dressed and ready to leave before you start getting the person in your care ready. It may be hard for him to wait for you.

- If the person in your care generally resists going to the doctor, do not talk about the appointment before you get there. Instead, talk about something pleasant that you are going to do together, such as having lunch at a restaurant or visiting a friend.

- Try to bring a family member, friend, or home health aide along. Another person can help you reassure or distract the person in your care.

- If the person in your care is in the moderate or moderately severe stage of AD, pack a bag with a change of clothes, incontinence products, and some activity to occupy him or her while you wait in the office. Just before you leave, add a snack and a drink to this bag.

Tip If going to the doctor tends to be a problem, don't mention the visit in advance.

NOTE Be sure shots for tetanus, flu, and pneumonia are up-to-date. For those on Medicare, flu and pneumonia shots are covered.

At the Doctor's Office

Because the person in your care has Alzheimer's disease you may have to:

- Tell the doctor what you hope and expect from the visit and any recommended treatment.

- If the doctor tells you to do something you know you can't do, such as give medication in the middle of the night, ask if there is another treatment and explain why.

- Insist on talking about the level of care that you believe is appropriate and that agrees with the care receiver's wishes.

- Ask about other options for tests, medications, and surgery.

- Ask why tests or treatments are needed and what the risks are.

- Consider all options, including the pros and cons of "watchful waiting."

- Trust your common sense and if you have doubts, get a second opinion.

 Tip Allow plenty of time to get to the appointment. People with AD cannot be rushed.

Dental Care

Dental care is important for overall wellness. For low-cost dental programs, check with university dental schools or the local Area Agency on Aging.

- Try to go to a dentist who knows how to work with people who have Alzheimer's disease.
- Ask if the office and dental chair are wheelchair accessible, if that is needed.
- Tell the dentist all the medications the person is taking before starting dental treatment.
- Find out how many visits will be needed.
- Ask about alternative options to the treatment that may be easy for the person with AD to tolerate.

Vision Care

A person with AD should have regular eye examinations. Poor vision can contribute to confusion. These exams can also spot or detect other serious diseases such as diabetes. Finding and treating eye disease early can prevent serious diseases from getting worse and leading to blindness.

- Tell the doctor of any medicines the person is taking.
- Tell the doctor if there is a family history of glaucoma.
- Get a yearly eye exam for a person with diabetes.

- Contact your state's Commission for the Blind for information on vision aids for those with low vision.

- Ask for help in finding products ("talking" watches, etc.) and aids that will help the person adjust to low vision.

- Seek out radio stations that have programs of newspaper readings if the person in your care is in the very early stage of AD.

Hearing

Hearing loss can make it more difficult for a person to understand and respond appropriately or take part in social activities. It will help the person to hear if you speak slowly and clearly, rather than raising your voice. It is difficult for anyone to adjust to a hearing aid, and more difficult for someone with AD, but it may be worth exploring the possibility of getting one.

Mental and Emotional Health

People with dementia often have emotional symptoms such as depression and anxiety. These symptoms may be a direct result of the neurological changes caused by the illness. They can also be the person's reaction to the *awareness* of change in his ability to function as he once could. In addition, depression and anxiety can be a symptom of another illness entirely or of medications used to treat it.

By keeping the person with AD *physically* healthy, you will be also helping him to maintain a positive emotional balance. Illness and pain, though sometimes unavoidable, can lead to a depressed and anxious mood. It is important to consult the person's doctor to find out whether there is a physical illness that might account for a sudden change in mood or other emotional symptoms.

A person in the early stage of Alzheimer's disease may still be able to express feelings of sadness, loss, hopelessness, or even to say that she feels depressed. Symptoms of depression include a loss of interest in activities and hobbies, not wanting to be with people, and irritability. There may also be some physical symptoms such as change in appetite, fatigue, and sleep problems, although these may also be symptoms of another medical condition. It is not easy to separate out the symptoms of Alzheimer's from those of depression and a person may have both illnesses.

As with any depressed person, it is not helpful to tell him "get with the program," "cheer up, things could be worse" or to "try harder." It is best to respond by providing more emotional support and meaningful activities and including him in family life as much as possible.

Symptoms of depression in people with Alzheimer's disease sometimes seem to come and go, unlike the cognitive (ability to think) problems that get worse over time. But if your efforts to relieve his negative mood do not work, he should be evaluated by a psychiatrist who specializes in the care of the elderly with dementia. An antidepresssant medication may help the person in your care feel better, but as with all medications, should be checked regularly to ensure that the drug is still helping and is not causing unacceptable side effects. Strong emotions are a normal part of long-term illness. Counseling and support groups are a very helpful way of dealing with these feelings. If the person with dementia is depressed and needs therapy, ask the primary care doctor to give you the name of a therapist.

How to Tell If a Person with Alzheimer's Disease Is in Pain

It can be difficult to figure out whether someone with dementia is in pain, and what is causing the pain. People with dementia may not be able to tell you in words that they are in pain, or even where the pain is. Sometimes they can be in great pain, and not be able to communicate directly.

In the early stage of dementia, she may answer in what seems like a response to the question the doctor is asking, even though she does not understand the question but is simply trying to be helpful. For example, wherever the doctor touches and asks, "Does it hurt here?" She may keep saying, "Yes." This does not help the doctor to figure out where the pain is.

You know the person in your care better than the doctor, so you will be able to interpret her way of communicating. Here are some signs of pain that will be of help when the person is unable to tell you directly—

- verbal cues—crying or moaning, calling out
- rubbing or protecting one part of the body
- facial expression, frowning, or grimacing
- decreased activity level
- trouble sleeping
- a stiffened upper or lower body that is held rigidly and moved slowly
- increased agitation, aggressive behavior, pacing or rocking
- mental status changes, increased confusion or irritability

Each person has his or her own *pain signature*. Because you know this person, you will know what behavior is typical. You can recognize that there is a change in behavior and perhaps when that change indicates pain.

What to Do in an Emergency

In the course of caring for a person with Alzheimer's disease it is likely that an accident will occur or that the person will appear to be seriously ill. A person with dementia can fall and break a bone, and not complain of pain. On the other hand, a relatively minor illness or discomfort may make the person extremely upset. Because of his dementia, the person may not be able to help you to decide what kind of care is needed. Is this an emergency? If it is, you should call 911, the fire department or whatever agency is in charge of sending the Emergency Medical Service in your area. You should not try to take the person to the emergency room on your own. How can you decide that there is an emergency? The following signs always indicate an emergency that needs immediate attention—

- loss of consciousness or a marked change in mental state
- sudden severe chest pain
- a fall that results in severe pain or inability to move
- an accident that results in a blow to the head
- uncontrollable bleeding
- high fever accompanied by confusion and delusions
- difficulty breathing
- repeated or forceful vomiting
- failure to urinate for more than twelve hours
- sudden slurring of speech, loss of vision or balance, extreme weakness
- violent or uncontrollable behavior
- swallowing a poisonous substance

From *The Alzheimer's Health Care Handbook,* Mittelman and Epstein, copyright 2003 by Mary S. Mittelman, DrPH.

Even if none of these signs are present and you think that the person is seriously ill, call for emergency help. No caregiver looks forward to a visit to the emergency room, but it is a better alternative than neglecting a situation that could be life threatening.

 If the person in your care is enrolled in a hospice program find out in advance what arrangements the program has for emergency care.

Under the stress of an emergency you don't want to be looking around for items you may need. It is best to put them all in one place in advance. Perhaps you can put them in a small suitcase. Include:

- Insurance documents, advance directives, and the Profile of the Person with Memory Impairment if it is filled out (see pp. 62–66)

- A list of the medications the person is taking

- A small notebook and a pen or pencil; once you are at the hospital, you will want to jot down names of doctors and other hospital personnel, procedures, questions and answers, and reminders to yourself and others

What else can you do while you are waiting for the ambulance to come?

- If you have a cellular phone, find it so you can take it along. If not, have lots of change or a telephone card for using the public phone.

- Make sure you have your own wallet, with identification, credit card, and some cash for food, reading material, other incidentals, and to pay for a taxi, which may be needed if the person in your care is able to go home instead of being admitted to the hospital.

- If the person with AD is not dressed, bring along a pair of shoes, clothes, and a coat to be worn home if he or she is not admitted to the hospital. Be sure not to bring valuables, such as expensive watches, rings, and other jewelry; and do not plan to leave more than a few dollars with him. An inexpensive watch is okay if he generally wears one at home.

- Let someone else in your family or a friend know that you are taking your relative to the hospital and could use a helping hand.

- If time permits call the person's doctor to let her know that you are taking the person in your care to the E.R.

Adapted from *The Alzheimer's Health Care Handbook*, Mittelman and Epstein, copyright 2003 by Mary S. Mittelman, DrPH.

 Tip
If the situation allows, ask that the person be taken to the hospital with which his doctor is affiliated to facilitate continuity of care.

Once you arrive in the emergency room do your best to stay with the person in your care and to inform all staff members that he has Alzheimer's disease and may not be able to provide accurate information about his condition or to follow their instructions.

 NOTE A major cause of emergency room visits for frail or demented older adults is dehydration.

Dehydration occurs when a person is either not getting enough liquids daily or excreting too much urine. The body's ability to detect thirst diminishes with age. Illness and medication can also cause dehydration. Signs and symptoms of dehydration include:

- Headache—the most common symptom
- Dry mouth and tongue
- Cracked lips
- Dry skin
- Sunken eyes
- Nausea, vomiting, diarrhea
- Dark, strong smelling urine
- Weight loss
- Fast heart beat
- Low blood pressure
- Confusion, light-headedness
- Disorientation

In the Hospital

Being in the hospital is especially difficult for someone with AD. You will have to make special efforts to keep the person in your care safe and comfortable in the hospital. While it may be best if you are there, you also need to take care of *yourself*. Find friends and relatives who can take your place at the bedside so you can get an occasional rest.

Let's consider how a hospital experience might feel for a person with Alzheimer's—

- he finds it stressful to be around strange people
- he becomes upset when his normal daily routine is disrupted—the patient is expected to adjust to the schedule of the hospital

- he may undergo painful treatments and examinations without understanding why

- he may misinterpret what is being done to him and feel attacked or threatened

- it is natural that a sick person will not handle stress well; when the person has dementia, his reactions are usually more extreme

It is not surprising that some people with Alzheimer's feel frightened, confused and agitated in the hospital. Because they may not understand what is happening to them, they may become aggressive and uncooperative.

Adapted from *The Alzheimer's Health Care Handbook,* Mittelman and Epstein, copyright 2003 by Mary S. Mittelman, DrPH.

Special Help

Be aware that a person with AD may need help with some basic activities that go on in the hospital. She may not be able to find the bathroom or realize that she needs help while there; it is best if she not go alone. She may not know how to use the call button or remember that it is there. She may not remember to follow dietary restrictions or know how to fill out the menu. She might need help eating. For reasons like these it is best if the person with AD has someone with him at the hospital as much as possible.

It is a good idea to speak with the nurse about the needs of the person in your care; give the nurse a copy of the **Profile of the Person with Memory Impairment** and let her know of your concerns.

If the person with AD is well enough to get up and walk around be careful that he not wander and get lost. Again, the best way to keep him safe is to keep him under supervision at all times. It is during the night that people with AD often need the most support. You may need to consider hiring help for the wee hours if no one is able to stay with the person overnight.

Tip Check to see that medications for Alzheimer's are still being administered, unless there is a medical reason to discontinue them. While they may not be a priority in terms of the acute illness that brought the person to the hospital, they are important for continued Alzheimer's care.

NOTE Remember, normal hospital procedures may feel like physical and emotional *assaults* to a person with Alzheimer's disease.

How to Watch Out for Someone's Best Interests in the Hospital

In the hospital a person with dementia is at greater risk than others, so be ready to keep tabs on treatments, ask questions, and act as an advocate.

- If the Patients' Bill of Rights is not posted in a place where it can be seen, ask for a copy.

- Agree only to treatments that have been thoroughly explained.

- If something is not being done and you think it should be, ask why.

- Be friendly and show respect to hospital staff. They will probably respond better to you and to the person in your care. Bad feelings between family members and staff may cause the staff to avoid the person.

- Assist with the person's grooming and care.

- Speak up if you notice doctors or nurses examining anyone without first washing their hands.

• Check all bills and ask questions about anything that isn't clear to you.

Reducing Stress in the Hospital

You can do a great deal to help reduce the stress the person with dementia is feeling. One of the most important things you can do is to stay with him as much as possible. *You* know best how to calm and communicate with him and can help the staff to understand his reactions.

Be sure to tell the hospital staff that your relative has dementia. Because information does not always get passed from shift to shift, you should tell any staff members you haven't seen before about his dementia and about what his normal behavior is like. Try to develop a working relationship with the staff so that your role of advocate (supporter) will be more effective.

NOTE As the caregiver to a person with AD, you have to be able to speak for the person with the hospital staff. Do not be afraid to ask for a second opinion. The doctors will understand that you need as much information as you can get when making decisions for someone else.

Let the staff know that you want to be regularly informed about the medical plan and the medications given to your care receiver. A person with Alzheimer's disease will not be able to know if he is getting the correct medication. Set up times to meet with the doctor so that you can get and give feedback on the person's progress. The hospital social worker will be able to help you make these arrangements.

Try to arrange a room in the quietest place on the floor. If he must share a room with another patient, explain to that person and his family that he has dementia and may not be able to follow the regular rules of etiquette. If the roommate has frequent visitors who upset the person in your care, it may be necessary to request a room or roommate change.

Tip

If you are having a problem in the hospital that you cannot resolve, you may get additional support from the Patient Representative. The representative will be familiar with hospital procedures and may be able to help you to get what you need or explain why it is not possible.

Throughout the course of the person's hospital stay, pay attention to *your* own level of stress and fatigue. If you don't get enough help from family and friends you may need to hire a professional aide. This can be done through the hospital.

When it is time to go home, a discharge planner should meet with you to develop a discharge plan. You may need to work to get the resources that will be needed to continue the person's recovery. Keep in mind that caregiving will be more difficult when he comes home and you will need your strength to meet these additional demands.

Occasionally people with dementia are hospitalized in the psychiatric ward of a hospital because their behavioral symptoms are getting worse in spite of dedicated and compassionate home care or medication. Many of the suggestions in this chapter will also be helpful in the psychiatric unit.

Checklist **A More Comfortable Hospital Stay**

These are some of the ways you can make the person with AD more comfortable in the hospital:

✓ Lower the ringers on the telephones.

✓ Ask that the intercom be used as little as possible.

✓ Change the lighting. Ask if a bright light can be left on near the patient if the person is afraid of shadows.

✓ Cover pictures.

✓ Limit the number of visitors.

✓ If the patient is upset by the view from the window, close the curtains.

✓ Look around and see how you can simplify the room. Ask what equipment can be removed or put away in the closets or hidden behind a curtain. Put items in drawers that the patient does not use all the time.

✓ Leave eyeglasses and other essentials within easy reach.

✓ If there is a wheelchair in the room for the patient, put it in the hall.

✓ If possible, push the bed against the wall so the patient can only get out on one side and you will have more room to move around.

✓ Close the curtain that surrounds the bed to make a more private space that may feel safer to the patient.

✓ When magazines, leftover juice and wilting flowers start to accumulate, make a clean sweep and put the room in order again.

(From *The Alzheimer's Health Care Handbook,* Mittelman and Epstein, copyright 2003 by Mary S. Mittelman, DrPH.)

According to federal law, a hospital must release patients in a *safe manner* or else must keep them in the hospital. Letting a patient leave the hospital is not wise if the person has constant fever, infection or pain that cannot be controlled, confusion and excess disorientation suggesting delirium, a common problem in people with dementia (no sense of time or place), or is unable to take food and liquids by mouth. However, in some cases, it may be better for the person to be released because the noise and risk of catching other diseases may make it more difficult to recover. If you plan to appeal a discharge, understand the rules of Medicare, Medicaid, the HMO, or insurance plan.

When You Doubt the Time Is Right for Discharge

- State your doubts in a simple letter to the hospital's director or the health plan's medical director. (Rules vary from state to state.)

- Meet with the hospital's discharge planner.

- Ask if the hospital is following the usual policy for the condition.

- Explain any special reasons that make you think it is unwise to discharge the person.

- Ask if the hospital rules can be changed to cover this special case.

- Remember that anyone has the right to appeal a discharge.

- Get your doctor's help in the appeal, but understand that he or she may have different reasons for wanting to discharge the person.

Sometimes hospitalization provides a chance for you to rethink the care plan for the person with dementia. If the level of dementia has increased as a result of the hospitalization, you will have to know what additional resources you need or other housing options you should consider.

Ask the social worker in the hospital to help you. The social worker is required to create a safe discharge plan. While you can express your thoughts and needs, the person's insurance coverage will probably be the most important factor in determining what services you will be offered.

Nursing Home Placement

At the end of a hospital stay, hospital staff frequently recommend nursing home placement, even if the family objects and wants to take the patient home. In some cases, the staff may realize that the caregiver is exhausted and may not be able to continue providing care. Before you reject nursing home placement for the person, honestly consider whether the time has come when this may be the safest, most reasonable choice.

Subacute Facility Placement

If the person requires physical rehabilitation or more care than can be offered comfortably and safely at home, but no longer needs hospitalization, a subacute facility is an option at discharge. These facilities may be located in nursing homes but are meant for short-term stays. This may be a very useful option but it may lead to cognitive and functional decline (loss of function) because the person with dementia will once again be in an unfamiliar place.

Consider the risks and benefits of the different care options. If you do decide to take the person home, it may be necessary to make changes to the home and the

Checklist **Coming Home from the Hospital**

✓ Assess the person's condition and needs.

✓ Understand the diagnosis (what is wrong) and prognosis (what will happen).

✓ Become part of the health care team (doctor, nurse, therapists) so you can learn how to provide care.

✓ Get complete written instructions from the doctor. If there is anything you don't understand, ASK QUESTIONS.

✓ Arrange follow-up care from the doctor.

✓ Develop a plan of care with the doctor. (See **Setting Up a Plan for Day-to-Day Activities, p. 139.**)

✓ Meet with the hospital's social worker or discharge planner to determine home care benefits.

✓ Understand in-home assistance options. (See **Hiring and Paying for Care, p. 57.**)

✓ Arrange for in-home help.

✓ Arrange physical, occupational, and speech therapy as needed.

✓ Find out if medicine is provided by the hospital to take home. If not, you will have to have prescriptions filled before you take the person home.

✓ Prepare the home. (See **Preparing the Home, p. 21.**)

✓ Buy needed supplies; rent, borrow, or buy equipment such as wheelchairs, crutches, and walkers.

✓ Take home all personal items.

✓ Check with the hospital cashier for discharge payment requirements.

✓ Arrange transportation (an ambulance or van if your car will not do).

care plan as well as to look into additional resources. It can be very difficult and stressful to try to learn to give some of the new treatments at home. There are agencies that provide nursing services at home. If equipment is needed, the company that provides it may also offer help in how to use it.

 NOTE Be Prepared! People with dementia often become more confused in the hospital because of the stress of an unfamiliar environment. If she is discharged home, she may get back to her old self with time. If she does not, you may need to consider a new plan of care.

When to Consider Hospice Care

AD is a progressive disease. If the person does not die of another condition, AD itself will cause his death. Hospice care can provide the comfort and support that the person with the illness and his family need during the last months of life. A person will go through many physical, emotional, and spiritual changes as death approaches.

What Hospice Care Will Provide

Hospice care is delivered by a team of specially trained medical professionals who focus on easing pain and managing symptoms. They provide medical, emotional, psychological, and spiritual care to the person and his family. They assist the family in coping with their coming loss and their grief afterward. Most hospice care is delivered in the home, but hospice care can also be provided in hospitals, nursing homes, and hospice facilities. The person who is ill and the family are the core of the hospice team and are at the center of all decision making.

Although a family member or other caregiver cares for the person on a daily basis, a hospice nurse is available 24 hours a day to provide advice and make visits. Hospice services include—

- physician services

- nursing services

- medical social services

- home health aide and homemaker services

- spiritual, dietary, and other counseling

- physical, occupational, and speech–language therapy

- medicine for controlling pain

- medical supplies and appliances

- ongoing care at home or in the hospital during periods of crisis

- special services for grief counseling

- trained volunteers for companionship, errands, or respite

- bereavement (grief) services for the family (or loved ones) for up to a year after death

Although the attending physician typically refers a person to hospice, a family member, friend, or caregiver may also contact the hospice.

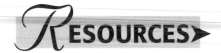

For free or low-cost resources, contact local consumer health resource and information centers (check the local hospital system or phone book) and local health agencies or associations (American Heart Association, American Diabetes Association, National Multiple Sclerosis Society, and others).

American Academy of Medical Acupuncture
www.medicalacupuncture.org
Will provide the names of member acupuncturists who are also medical doctors.

Doctor's Guide to the Internet—Patient Edition
www.pslgroup.com/PTGUIDE.HTM
Provides information for specific diseases and gives pointers to other Internet sites of medical information.

Go Ask Alice!
www.goaskalice.columbia.edu/about.html
Provides helpful information and lets you post health-related questions.

The Health Resource, Inc.
933 Faulkner Street
Conway, AR 72034
(800) 949-0090; (501) 329-5272; Fax (501) 329-9489
www.thehealthresource.com
Provides clients with personalized detailed reports on their specific medical conditions. These reports contain conventional and alternative treatments and information on current research, nutrition, self-help measures, specialists, and resource organizations. Reports on any non-cancer condition are $295, or $395 for complex issues, and contain 50 to 100 pages. Reports on any cancer condition are $395 and contain 150 to 200 pages. Shipping is additional.

Hospice Foundation of America
2001 S Street NW, #300
Washington, DC 20009
Tel: (800) 854-3402
Provides information and referral service, resources on end-of-life care, a search engine to end-of-life Web sites, free brochures on hospice, volunteering, and bereavement.

How to Care
www.howtocare.com

The National Chronic Pain Outreach Association
P.O. Box 274
Millboro, VA 24460
(540) 862-9437
Fax: (540)862-9485
www.chronicpain.org
E-mail: ncpoa@cfw.com
A membership organization that offers a quarterly newsletter (Lifeline), a catalogue of related publications, national physician referrals, and support group listings. Membership is $25 per year.

University of Washington
www.uwmedicine.org
A great storehouse of general health information on all topics.

The Worldwide Congress on Pain
http://www.pain.com

Information About Eyesight

Lighthouse International
111 E. 59th Street
New York, NY 10022
(800) 829-0500
www.lighthouse.org

Lions Club International
300 W. 22nd Street
Oak Brook, IL 60523
www.lionsclub.org
(630) 571-5466

National Association for Visually Handicapped
22 West 21st Street, 6th floor
New York, NY 10010
(212) 889-3141
www.navh.org

National Federation of the Blind
1800 Johnson Street
Baltimore, MD 21230
(410) 659-9314
www.nfb.org

Medications

Together Rx Access™ Card
A joint program by drug companies offering a free Prescription Savings Card for individuals and families who meet all four of the following requirements:

❏ *Not eligible for Medicare*

❏ *Have no public or private prescription drug coverage*

❏ *Household income equal to or less than:*
—*$30,000 for a single person*
—*$40,000 for a family of two*
—*$50,000 for a family of three*
—*$60,000 for a family of four*
—*$70,000 for a family of five*

❏ *Legal resident of the U.S. or Puerto Rico*

Call 1-800-250-2839 to start saving on your prescriptions. For the most current list of medicines and products, visit www.TogetherRxAccess.com

Publications

A Family Caregiver's Guide to Hospital Discharge Planning, a publication of the National Alliance for Caregiving and the United Hospital Fund of New York. Available at www.caregiving.org

The Alzheimer's Health Care Handbook, by M. Mittelman & C. Epstein. Marlowe and Company. New York, 2003.
A comprehensive resource on providing medical care.

The Comfort of Home™:A Complete Guide for Caregivers, by Meyer & Derr. CareTrust Publications, 2007.
Provides a complete list of questions to ask to ask before agreeing to tests, surgery, medications, and more.

If you don't have access to the Internet, ask your local library to help you locate a Web site.

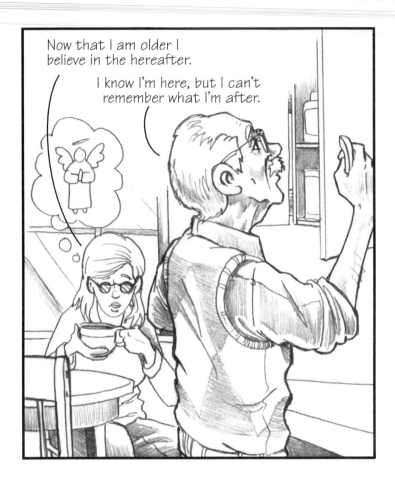

A person without a sense of humor is like a wagon without wheels—jolted by every pebble in the road.

—Henry Ward Beecher

Part Two: Day-by-Day Living with Alzheimer's Disease

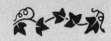

Setting Up a Plan for Day-to-Day Activities

Setting Up a Plan for Day-to-Day Activities

*O*ne of the results of Alzheimer's disease is that the person is unable to plan how to spend her time. She is also unlikely to initiate activities and reach out to friends or family. She often spends much of the day napping and pacing, which results in what others would judge to be an "empty day." She may also forget to have meals, toilet herself, and conduct other routine activities. That is why it is important for you to set up a plan for day-to-day activities that can be followed on a regular basis. In time, the person will become familiar with the routine you have set up, and will feel reassured by knowing what to expect. When you need to change the plan, for special occasions or unusual occurrences, try to go back to the regular routine as soon as possible. In the early stage of AD, people may need to have activities suggested to them, and be reminded to take medications on schedule and to keep important appointments. In the middle stage, a more formal structure should be established by the caregiver. In the late stage, the routine will have to be modified to take into account the person's declining functional abilities, remembering the remaining strengths. A typical daily schedule for a person in the middle stage of AD follows.

Meaningful Activities

The work we do and the activities we choose for fun tell the world a lot about us. Try to imagine your life without them. People with Alzheimer's disease lose the ability to do the things that make them who they are little by little over time.

It is common for caregivers to focus on the activities they need to stop the person with AD from doing, such as driving, working, going out alone, and making important decisions. However, in order to help the person maintain good self-esteem, it is important to also think about how to help him to continue to engage in meaningful activities, and participate in family and community life. To do this you need to decide what type of things he can do and help him adjust for abilities that are lost. As the old song says, you need to "accentuate the positive."

Think about ways the person can continue to participate in activities she enjoyed before becoming ill. For example, if she used to play tennis, but can no longer keep score, would she enjoy hitting the ball back and forth? If she enjoyed cooking, can you and she make a meal together? Can she stir a sauce if you watch to be sure she doesn't get burned?

Activities give structure to time. They should make the best use of a person's remaining strengths and skills and be based on interests and hobbies that have been developed over a lifetime. They can include activities that you did together, such as going for walks or gardening, which can still be enjoyed. Meaningful activities can also reduce the risk that that the person will become agitated or behave in ways that may upset him and others. People with dementia have difficulty planning and in choosing activities. When a person is in the early stage, just a reminder or a cue may be enough to get him going and he may be able to carry on from there. But eventually you will have to do more. You will have to choose the

activity and create the physical and emotional environment in which the person with dementia can do it.

Without guidance, the person in your care may experience what is called the *empty-day syndrome*. Although people with Alzheimer's may not realize that they
are bored, they may just doze or become restless and
wander aimlessly about the house.

> *Tip*   Like anyone else, people with Alzheimer's disease are
> more likely to feel good about themselves if they
> engage in activities that stimulate and satisfy them.

Example of a Daily Schedule for a Person with Middle-Stage Alzheimer's Disease

TIME	ACTIVITY	NOTES
7:30 AM	Morning wake-up routine	Toileting or changing of incontinence products
7:45	BREAKFAST	Give morning medications
8:30	MORNING BATHROOM ROUTINE	Toileting, bath or shower, if typically done in the morning, brush teeth, etc.
9:00	GET DRESSED	
9:30	Go for a walk, visit with neighbor/family, exercise	If person does not attend day care
10:30	SNACK	Encourage fluids
11:00	BATHROOM BREAK	Change incontinence product
11:20	REST	

TIME	ACTIVITY	NOTES
12:00	LUNCH	
1:00	LISTEN TO MUSIC	
1:30	BATHROOM BREAK	
1:50	Go out to beauty parlor/barber*—outside activity–drive in the car *	If person can still enjoy this type of experience
3:30	SNACK	
4:00	BATHROOM BREAK	
4:20	RESPITE VIDEO/SORTING CARDS	If person is overstimulated, try a quiet activity/understimulated, try more engaging activity–i.e., puzzle, game
5:15	WASH UP FOR DINNER	
5:30	DINNER	Give evening medication
6:30	Relaxing evening activity—reading, coloring, watching television	
7:00	EVENING BATHROOM ROUTINE, including toileting	Shower/bath if not done in AM
7:30	CHANGE CLOTHING FOR BEDTIME	If person resists, let them sleep in day clothes
8:00	BEDTIME	

*These are suggested daily activities.

It is best to establish a routine that includes a balance of rest and activity. We recommend regularly changing incontinence products or encouraging a visit to the bathroom before leaving the house.

> **NOTE** Some people with AD get very upset watching violence on TV becasue they think it is real. Careful monitoring of the TV is important.

Finding an Activity

You don't need to think of an activity as something out of the ordinary. In fact, many regular activities of daily life can be modified so that the person with dementia can still do them.

Chores such as dusting, sweeping, doing laundry, preparing food, and cooking can be satisfying activities. Even bathing, shaving, and getting dressed can provide an opportunity for chatting and reminiscing, singing or telling jokes. Making these necessary daily activities enjoyable will probably help the person in your care to cooperate with the task so you both can enjoy it.

Make Activities More Fun

Don't tell the person about something you have planned for the future too soon before it is to happen. This may only cause anxiety, not pleasant expectation.

People with Alzheimer's disease have trouble concentrating. That means the person may not be able to continue to pay attention to a task without getting distracted. What were once simple tasks will take longer.

To figure out what activities the care receiver can still participate in, ask yourself: What did she used to enjoy? Is there a way to modify the activity so it is safe, and she can still enjoy it? She may enjoy attending religious services, and may find that she can perform some volunteer activity in her house of worship.

Don't be afraid to try something the person has not done before. As people age their interests may change and in spite of Alzheimer's or sometimes because of it, people discover talents they may not have expressed before such as painting or collage or even a greater sense of spirituality.

Tip Recognize the limitations of this person. Don't try the impossible! Long trips, 3-act plays, a seat in the balcony far from the restroom are going to cause both of you trouble. If the person in care has physical limitations, either because of age, frailty, other illnesses, or hearing or vision problems, the activity may need to be altered to make it possible for him to participate.

Whatever activity you try, think about where it will take place and whether the person with AD will be interested in participating. Sometimes if you start to do something he will want to join you.

Indoors, be sure there will be enough light, table space, protection for furniture and carpet. If you are planning an activity outside, pay attention to the weather and have alternative plans for rain, excessive heat or cold, etc.

Break the activity down into simple steps. Have all the necessary equipment at hand. Choose an activity that can be completed in a relatively short time. The process of the activity is more important than the product. It may be just as much fun to make mashed potatoes as a perfect soufflé.

Be generous with your praise of his efforts and do not criticize or correct when mistakes are made. You may want to lend a hand if some aspect of the activity is too difficult or time-consuming for him.

Try not to get upset if the person gets up and walks away in the middle of the project. People with Alzheimer's easily get distracted and tired. He may wander back and continue working or may get involved in something else.

Try to keep your sense of humor when the person in your care eats all the string beans that were supposed to be for dinner or licks the icing off the cake or folds the dirty laundry. That's Alzheimer's for you! Alzheimer's is not funny, but amusing things do happen.

AD Limitations and Tips

Problem	Tip
Poor memory	Focus on the present. *Today is a sunny day rather than do you remember that winter snowstorm?*
Talking about the past	Use this opportunity to learn about the past (as the person currently remembers it)
Difficulty with orientation to time and place	Provide cues such as pictures of a toilet on the bathroom door or symbols such as a spoon glued to kitchen door to help the person find his way around the house
Doesn't understand what to do	Simplify the instructions and speak slowly. *Show* what is to be done.

Not paying attention	Perhaps he is tired, or the activity is not interesting, too difficult, or confusing; try at a later time.
The job does not get done	Do not focus on the product. Keep reminding yourself it is not important.
The person with AD does it wrong	Keep your sense of humor!

Activity Checklist

Consider the following possibilities for activities the person with dementia may enjoy—

- Creative activities such as painting, playing the piano, and using materials such as Playdough (if the person will not try to eat it)
- Cognitive activities such as reading a book, looking at a magazine, doing crossword puzzles
- Spiritual activities such as praying and singing a hymn
- Spontaneous activities such going out to dinner or to visit friends
- Work-related: things such as making notes, typing, or organizing coupons and other papers
- Simple household chores
      Dusting
      Drying dishes
      Helping to cook or prepare meals
      Doing the laundry
      Organizing papers
      Shining shoes

Shredding papers for recycling
- Simple physical activities
  - Going for a walk
  - Doing exercises
  - Raking leaves
  - Playing catch
- Musical activities
  - Dancing
  - Listening to favorite music
  - Singing old favorite songs together
- Attending church services
- Visiting friends or family
- Playing board games and cards
- Using a workshop and tools (make sure it is safe)
- Watching television (unless the person becomes confused or upset) or respite videos (📖 see *Resources*, p. 150).

There are many activities that encourage non-verbal (using body language, movement, etc.) emotional expression. For example, caring for plants or pets can help the person with AD to express feelings of caring. She will still appreciate signs of affection. Depending on your relationship, holding hands, hugging, brushing hair, rubbing on hand cream or other adult uses of touch (acceptable adult expressions of caring and concern) may provide emotional satisfaction to both of you.

While you may enjoy expressing your own creativity in devising activities for the care receiver, there are also some "ready made" resources. There are catalogues with activities especially designed for people with dementia as well as videos in which the viewer is invited to interact with the person on the screen as well as music and subjects that may remind the person of earlier times. These are for people in the later stages and you want to be careful not to use materials that look too childlike. However, simple puzzles, sorting, matching, and stacking blocks or shapes can be appropriate for people with dementia. As always, safety is a prime concern and games that have small pieces or that can be swallowed or that have sharp edges should be avoided.

 Some people enjoy making simple pottery out of clay or homemade flour dough. Shapes can be cut from the dough with cookie cutters. Stamps made with a stamp pad produce instant art and can be an enjoyable repetitive activity. Using a pencil or crayon, tracing around geometric shapes or around a person's hand is a common project for children and can work for you. Some people enjoy doodling on a blank piece of paper. Keep in mind the capabilities of the person in your care and offer gentle encouragement.

Favorite Golden Oldies

Singing is an easy pastime that can be enjoyed anywhere. The following songs are familiar to most seniors and have melodies that are easy for sing-alongs.

- Let Me Call You Sweetheart
- Down by the Old Mill Stream
- You Are My Sunshine
- Yes! We Have No Bananas
- Daisy Bell (Daisy Daisy)
- Clementine
- He's Got the Whole World in His Hands
- Skip to My Lou
- Yankee Doodle
- God Bless America

> **Tip** Doing activities or chores that recall a person's work-related past can change sadness to happiness.

The Power of Choice

Dementia can strip individuals of their ability to control their world. Small choices, then, become very important. The more choices they can make for themselves, the more control they feel. And the more control they feel, the greater the sense of independence and self-esteem they enjoy.

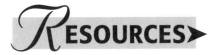

ElderSongPublications
P. O. Box 74
Mt. Airy, MD 21771
(800) 397-0533 Fax: (301) 829-5249
info@eldersong.com
http://nihseniorhealth.gov/alzheimerscare/
dailyactivities/02.html
Publisher of books, videos, and recordings for caregivers who work with older adults.

Nasco catalogue
ENASCO.com
901 Janesville Avenue
P.O. Box 901
Fort Atkinson, WI 53538-0901
800-558-9595 Fax: 920-563-8296
Art supplies and educational materials.

If you don't have access to the Internet, ask your local library to help you locate a Web site.

How to Avoid Caregiver Burnout

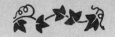

How to Avoid Caregiver Burnout

Stress occurs as a result of too many pressures that demand too much of you. The stress of caregiving can be overwhelming when you feel you have too many responsibilities and not enough support. If you feel very guilty, resentful, sad, and frightened or just in over your head all the time, your stress level will be high. It is natural for caregivers to experience these feelings from time to time. If you develop ways of coping with the demands of caregiving, and are aware of your level of stress, you will know when to seek more help, information, or time off. When you do not pay attention to your level of stress, you may ask more of yourself then you can give. If this "wear and tear" continues, you may become depressed, ill, isolated, and unable to provide care for the person with dementia or yourself.

Caregivers are frequently told to take care of themselves; they can offer a thousand reasons why they do not have the time, energy, money, etc. to do so. Be aware of your own excuses—whether real or imagined—against taking this advice. Think of ways you can incorporate some of the following to comfort yourself: prayer, talking with friends or relatives, exercise, hobbies, meditation, mindful breathing, yoga, walking, and seeking professional help or counseling. It is important to get help and support from other family members. Find a way to get respite from caregiving before you reach the point when you feel your life is out of control—burned out.

Burnout: Are You Suffering From It?

Often caregivers are not even aware that they are suffering from burnout until a friend or family member points out that they are not themselves. Caregivers can underestimate the impact of the work they are doing and the time and emotional energy they are using. Try not to be offended, but listen if you are told that you are more irritable than usual, seem to be losing your temper with the person you are caring for, and do not appear to be doing well.

Burnout may have some of the same symptoms as depression but is not the same and cannot be helped with medication. Burnout may explain your loss of interest in activities you used to enjoy, your run-down condition, feelings of hopelessness and helplessness, even wanting to hurt yourself or the person you are caring for. If you have these feelings it is time to re-evaluate your caregiving situation. You should take steps to get more support and relief from the constant responsibility and stress of caring for a person with Alzheimer's disease.

Where to Find Help

Are you feeling that you cannot or do not want to continue caregiving but that you have no choice but to keep going? The following suggestions may be of help.

- You may not be able to sort out this sensitive issue on your own. Find someone, a friend or counselor, who can listen and give you new ideas and perspective.

- Attend conferences and lectures about Alzheimer's disease or join a support group with other people who are going through the same thing.

- Hire more help or enlist more family involvement.

- Consider enrolling the person in your care in an adult day care program.

- Consider placing him in a residential care facility for a short stay while you take a vacation.

Caregiver Burnout Checklist:

Ask yourself the following questions:

	Yes	No
• What are your expectations? Are they realistic? Are you expecting the person with AD to get better or to always be pleasant because of all the time and concern you put into his care?	___	___
• Do you wish he would show gratitude?	___	___
• When expected help does not come through, do you get disappointed and try to do everything yourself?	___	___
• Are you feeling tired, isolated, helpless, angry, resentful, or guilty?	___	___
• Are you physically ill yourself and not going to the doctor or following the doctor's instructions about how to care for yourself?	___	___
• Have you stopped making time for yourself, to refuel and nourish your own interests and friendships?	___	___
• Are you using destructive ways of coping, such as alcohol, overeating, or misusing drugs?	___	___
• Have you caught yourself calling the person in your care bad names?	___	___
• Do you want to scream at him?	___	___
• Are you afraid you may hurt him?	___	___

- Seriously consider whether you want to continue providing hands-on care. Both you and the person with AD may do better if he is placed in a care facility. You then may be able to visit, to keep an eye on the care, and to enjoy being together when you are no longer the front-line person.

Emotional Burdens

You may think you are the only one to face these problems, but you are not alone. Many caregivers face—

- the need to hide their grief
- fear of the future
- worries about money
- not being able to solve problems

Dependency and Isolation

Fears of dependency and loneliness, or isolation, are common in families of those who are ill. The person needing care can become more and more dependent on the one who is providing it. At the same time, the caregiver needs others for respite and support. Many caregivers are ashamed about needing help, so they don't ask for it. Those caregivers who are able to develop personal and social support have a greater sense of well-being.

 Spouse caregivers have special problems as they gradually lose the emotional support of the partner who is ill and must now be his or her emotional as well as physical support. It is especially important for spouse caregivers to seek out a support system.

"**Why doesn't anyone ask how I am doing?**" It is easy to feel invisible, as if no one can see you. Everyone's attention is on the person with the illness, and they don't seem to understand what the caregiver is going through. Many caregivers say that nobody even asks how they're doing. Mental health experts say it's not wise to let feelings of neglect build up. Caregivers need to speak up and tell other people what they need and how they feel.

Support groups, religious or spiritual advisors, or mental health counselors can teach you new and positive ways to express your own need for help.

Seek out professional help when you:

- are using more alcohol than usual to relax

- are using too many prescription medications

- have physical symptoms such as skin rashes, backaches, or a cold or flu that won't go away

- are unable to think clearly or focus

- feel tired and don't want to do anything

- feel keyed up and on edge

- feel sad all the time

- feel intense fear and anxiety

- feel worthless and guilty

- are depressed for two weeks or more

- are having thoughts of suicide

- have become or are thinking about becoming physically violent toward the person you are caring for

Before Hostility Builds to the Breaking Point

Anger and frustration *must* be addressed and healthy outlets found as a way to let off steam. If they are not, angry situations can become physically or emotionally abusive. (See *Abuse and Neglect*, p. 159).

If you cannot control your emotions, try to find a safe way to release them.

- Take a walk or get some exercise to cool down.

- Write your thoughts in a journal.

- Go to a private corner and take out your anger on a big pillow.

> **NOTE** You cannot leave a person with AD alone if he is beyond the early stage of the illness. You will need to find someone else to step in temporarily when you leave.

Negative Emotions That You May Feel

The challenges of the caregiver role may sometimes make you feel bad about yourself. If you are a perfectionist, you'll never do it perfectly. If you're angry, you'll find plenty of excuses to be mad. If you have feelings of inadequacy, they'll definitely come up. Impatience, depression, hostility—if these emotions challenged you before, they're sure to arise in this situation.

Guilt Can Be Crippling

You can easily believe that you're not doing a good-enough job as caregiver. Keep in mind that you are doing the best you can, and stay open to suggestions that can help you improve.

Depression Is Dangerous

Depression endangers your own health and well-being and your ability to provide care.

Symptoms of Depression

Here are the symptoms:

- persistent sad, anxious or "empty" mood
- feelings of hopelessness, pessimism
- feelings of guilt, worthlessness, helplessness
- loss of interest or pleasure in hobbies and activities that were once enjoyed, including sex
- decreased energy, fatigue, being "slowed down"
- difficulty concentrating, remembering, making decisions
- insomnia, early-morning awakening, or oversleeping
- appetite and/or weight changes
- thoughts of death or suicide, or suicidal attempts
- restlessness, irritability

If you have five or more of these symptoms for longer than two weeks, depression may be the cause. Talk to a physician, psychiatrist, social worker, or psychologist about treatment options. The most effective treatment combines medication with talking therapy. Your well-being is as important as that of the person in our care.

- Claim time for yourself and make sure you use it.
- Make and keep doctor's appointments for yourself.
- Join a caregiver support group.
- Take advantage of respite care opportunities.

Anger

It is easy to feel victimized in this situation; you are caught up in the problems caused by someone else's illness. One natural response is anger. Unleashing anger on the person in your care may make you feel guilty that you have expressed anger; think of it as a message to yourself that you need more respite or support. Try these outlets:

- Caregiver support groups provide a place where you can freely express your feelings. Everyone there understands; no one will make you feel guilty. Members will often offer effective, real-world solutions.

- Make an appointment with a therapist or family counselor or clergyperson.

- Keep a journal of your feelings.

- Separate the person from the condition. The illness, not the person in your care, is responsible for the difficulties and challenges that you both are facing. Don't blame the care receiver for the situation you are in.

- You may wish that you could explain to the person with AD how hard you are trying, and that he would express understanding and appreciation. Unfortunately, the ability to do this may be lost, for the person may not be able to find the words. You can share these feelings and needs with others who are able to respond.

Abuse and Neglect

Elder abuse can involve any of the following—

- physical abuse
- psychological/emotional abuse
- financial abuse
- neglect
- abandonment

You may find it difficult to imagine that the words "abuse" and "neglect" could be used to describe the way you treat the person in your care—whether he is a relative, friend, or client. Most caregivers do their best to care for their relatives, but abuse and neglect do happen.

If you feel that you are at the end of your rope, and have caught yourself using force to get him to do something he is resisting, or slapped him, that is called physical abuse. If you do not provide adequate food or water (unless the person is at the end of life and in hospice care) or needed assistance with activities of daily living, such as maintaining personal hygiene, that is considered neglect.

People with Alzheimer's disease can become physically or verbally abusive as part of the disease. They cannot help themselves, but that does not give their caregivers permission to abuse them. This may be very difficult to accept if you don't keep in mind the fact that the disease is causing the person to behave this way. You do not have the same excuse.

People with dementia are especially vulnerable to mistreatment, partly because caring for them can put so much stress on those who provide care. If you don't understand the reason for his behavior, you may misinterpret it as hostile to you, rather than caused by their illness. Understanding the disease, knowing how best to communicate with a person with dementia, and having iadequate support for yourself can go a long way toward preventing these very upsetting situations.

Signs of Elder Abuse

Knowing the signs and symptoms of abuse can help you determine if there is a problem. Signs and symptoms may include—

- Physical injury—bruises, cuts, burns or rope marks, broken bones or sprains that can't be explained.

- Emotional abuse—if the person you are caring for expresses feelings of helplessness, a hesitation to talk openly, fear, withdrawal, depression, or agitation.

- Lack of physical care—malnourishment, weight loss, poor hygiene, as well as bedsores, soiled bedding, unmet medical needs.

- Unusual behaviors—changes in the person's behavior or emotional state such as withdrawal, fear, or anxiety, apathy.

- Changes in living arrangements without notifying anyone.

- Unexplained changes such as the appearance of previously uninvolved relatives or newly met strangers moving in.

- Financial changes—missing money or valuables, unexplained financial transactions, unpaid bills despite available funds, and sudden transfer of assets.

Be alert to the senior's comments about being taken advantage of, but be aware that a person with AD may not be an accurate reporter.

 If you feel that you or a family member is either abusing or neglecting a person with Alzheimer's call the Alzheimer's Association 24-hour help line **1-800-272-3900**.

What You Can Do If You Suspect Someone Else Is Abusing the Person in Your Care

If the person you suspect is a paid employee, first report the problem to the agency. If you have hired the person privately, fire her. If the abuse is severe enough, report it to the police. If the person you suspect is a family member who has significant responsibility for care, try to find alternative care for the person with dementia. Ultimately, you can call Adult Protective Services or the police. The Adult Protective Services Agency—a part of the human service agency in most states—is usually responsible for investigating reports of domestic elder abuse and providing families with help and guidance. Other professionals who may be able to help include doctors or nurses, police officers, lawyers, and social workers.

 NOTE If someone you care about is in imminent danger, **call 911** or the police.

Out-of-State Calls

If your concern is for someone who lives in another state, call the Eldercare Locator [(800) 677-1116] for the in-state phone number. The people who staff the locator can help you to find assistance. All these hotlines are free and anonymous.

NOTE As many as 1.2 million seniors have been abused at some point in their lives. Those most at risk of being abused are people who suffer from dementia.
(Source: American Geriatrics Society)

Where to Find Professional Help or Support Groups

- the local chapter of the Alzheimer's Association
- the community pages of the phone directory

- the local county medical society, which can provide a list of counselors, psychologists, and psychiatrists

- religious service agencies

- community health clinics

- religious and spiritual advisors

- United Way's "First Call for Help"

- a hospital's social service department

- a newspaper calendar listing of support group meetings

- Area Agency on Aging

Ask for help from a counselor who is familiar with the needs of caregivers.

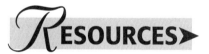

RESOURCES

Caregiver Survival Resources
www.caregiver911.com
A comprehensive list linking caregiving information and services for general issues and specific chronic illnesses.

Caregiver.com
www.caregiver.com
Maintains one of the most visited caregiver sites on the Internet. Publishes Today's Caregiver Magazine. *Provides links to many resources such as government and nonprofit agencies.*

Center for Family Caregivers/Tad Publishing Co.
www.caregiving.com or www.familycaregivers.org
Develops and distributes educational materials on caregiving, including a newsletter. Caregiving informational kits are $5 each; please specify new, seasoned, or transitioning caregiver when requesting a kit.

Eldercare Locator
(800) 677-1116
www.eldercare.gov
The local AAA is one of the first resources a family caregiver for an adult 60 years or older should contact when help is needed. Almost every state has one or more AAA, which serves local communities, older residents, and their families. Local AAAs are generally listed in the city or county government sections of the telephone directory under "Aging" or "Social Services." A caregiver can identify the nearest AAA by contacting the Eldercare Locator.

Lotsa Helping Hands
www.lotsahelpinghands.com
Provides a free-of-charge Web service that allows family, friends, neighbors, and colleagues to assist more easily with daily meals, rides, shopping, baby-sitting, and errands that may become a burden during times of medical crisis.

National Alliance for Caregiving
4720 Montgomery Lane, 5th Floor
Bethesda, MD 20184
www.caregiving.org
The Alliance is a non-profit coalition of national organizations focusing on issues of family caregiving.

National Family Caregivers Association
10400 Connecticut Avenue, Suite 500
Kensington, MD 20895
(800) 896-3650
info@thefamilycaregiver.org
www.thefamilycaregiver.org
Free member benefits include Take Care!, *a quarterly newsletter;* The Resourceful Caregiver, *a useful guide to resources; a support hotline and online chat room.*

Today's Caregiver Magazine
6365 Taft Street, Suite 3003
Hollywood, FL 33024
(800) 829-2734
www.caregiver.com/magazine
Bimonthly magazine dedicated to caregivers.

Well Spouse Association
63 West Main Street, Suite H
Freehold, NJ 07728
(800) 838-0879
info@wellspouse.org
www.wellspouse.org
Publishes Mainstay, *a bimonthly newsletter and provides networking/local support groups.*

See p. 251 for more Alzheimer's Caregiver Organizations.

Check with your local church or health facility to see if they sponsor **Share the Care** teams.

Publications

A Caregiver's Survival Guide: How to Stay Healthy When Your Loved One Is Sick, by Kay Marshall Strom. Intervarsity Press, 2000.

Care for the Family Caregiver: A Place to Start, a report prepared by HIP Health Plan of New York and National Alliance for Caregiving. Available at www.caregiving.org

Caring for Yourself While Caring for Others: A Caregiver's Survival and Renewal Guide, by Lawrence M. Brammer. Vantage Press, 1999.

Caring for Yourself While Caring for Your Aging Parents: How to Help, How to Survive, by Claire Berman. Henry Holt, 1996.

Helping Yourself Help Others: A Book for Caregivers, by Rosalynn Carter, with Susan Golant. Random House/Time Books, 1995.
Plenty of basic information for caregivers.

A Family Caregiver Speaks Up: It Doesn't Have to Be This Hard, by Suzanne Geffen Mintz. Capital Books, 2007.

Mainstay: For the Well Spouse of the Chronically Ill, by Maggie Strong.

Positive Caregiver Attitudes by James Sherman, PhD.

The Emotional Survival Guide for Caregivers by Barry J. Jacobs, PsyD. The Guilford Press, 2006.

The Fearless Caregiver: How to Get the Best Care From Your Loved One and Still Have a Life of Your Own, by Gary Barg. Capital Books, 2001.

If you don't have home access to the Internet, ask your local library to help you locate any Web site.

Understanding and Improving Communication

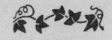

Understanding and Improving Communication

*C*ommunication *refers to the ability to speak, understand speech, read, write, and gesture. It is how we make contact with each other. Nonverbal messages are given through silence, body movements, or facial expression. As much as 90 percent of our communication is nonverbal. Be aware that words can carry one message and the body another; people with dementia seem to be especially sensitive to the* tone *or feeling of your communication and that is what they will react to.*

"Aphasia" (a-fā-zha) is a word for problems with language: it can affect speaking, understanding speech, reading, and writing. Aphasia is one of the problems associated with Alzheimer's disease. In the early stages of the disease, people have trouble thinking of common words while speaking or writing. In time, the ability to understand what others are saying also declines. While people with AD continue to be able to read, they eventually do not understand what they are reading. Communication problems get progressively worse over the course of the illness, until verbal communication becomes virtually impossible.

How to Be Understood

Tips for better communication—

• Keep good eye contact.

• Don't interrupt or distract the person while he is talking.

• Avoid criticizing, correcting and arguing.

- Focus on the feelings, not the facts. Sometimes the emotions being expressed are more important than what is being said. Look for the feelings behind the words.

- Always approach the person from the front. Tell the person who you are.

- Call the person by name. It helps orient the person and gets her attention.

- Use short, simple words and sentences. Talk slowly and clearly.

- Ask one question at a time.

- Give simple short explanations.

- Patiently wait for a response. A person may need extra time to process your request.

- Repeat information and questions. If the person doesn't respond, wait a moment. Then ask again. Perhaps if you rephrase and use other words, the person will understand better.

- Avoid quizzing. Reminiscing can be healthy, but avoid asking, "Do you remember when...?" Stay away from saying things like, "You should know who that is..."

- Break down tasks and instructions into clear, simple steps. Give one step at a time.

- Avoid confusing expressions. If you ask the person to "Hop in!" He or she may take that as a literal instruction. Describe the action directly to prevent confusion. "Please come here. Your shower is ready."

- Avoid vague words. Instead of saying "Here it is!"—try saying "Here is your hat."

- Turn negatives into positives. Instead of saying, "Don't go there," try saying, "Lets go to the dining room."

- Give visual cues. To help demonstrate the task, while asking him to do the task, point or touch the item you want the person to use. Or, begin the task for the person.

Source: Adapted from Teepa Snow, MS, OTR/L, FAOTA, Eastern North Carolina Alzheimer's Association Caregiver Training Programs, revised 2006.

 The most important thing to remember is to treat the person with dignity and respect. Avoid talking down to the person or talking to others as if he or she is not there. **At all times be aware of your tone of voice and body language.** Do not use the kind of high pitch that people sometimes use in speaking to children. Try to lower your pitch and sound and to be relaxed. Try not to be bossy or intimidating or stand over the person if he is sitting down. The person in your care may not understand your words, but he may nevertheless respond to the tone of your voice or your posture and will intuitively decide whether to respond to you as friend or foe.

Communication Problems at Each Stage of Alzheimer's Disease

People with Alzheimer's disease gradually have more and more trouble using and understanding words.

Early Stage

In the early stages, people with Alzheimer's disease may—

- Have difficulty finding the right word to say
- Use familiar words repeatedly
- Lose their train of thought

- Have difficulty following conversations when there are many speakers

- Have trouble with abstract terms–such as "his" or "her"

- Take long pauses between words

Since memory for recent events has declined, they may repeat themselves because they don't remember that they already have said something.

Helping the Person Communicate in the Early Stage of Alzheimer's Disease

There are many ways in which you can help a person in the early stage to continue to have the confidence to use his remaining verbal skills. You may ask if he wants you to suggest the word he cannot find or to remind him of what he was trying to say when he loses his trend of thought. If he is open to that kind of support, provide the missing word or connection without making an issue and let the conversation continue. If the person prefers to give himself time to come up with the missing word or idea on his own, wait patiently, and again, don't make a big deal, even if you feel impatient.

 One of the biggest challenges to caregivers or family members is to remain patient while coping with the changes in communication. The challenge will increases as the disease progresses.

Middle Stage

In the middle stages, people have more trouble expressing their feelings and needs with words.

- They may have trouble sticking to a subject or may even forget what they were intending to say.

- They may talk around a word they cannot remember; they will say, "You know the thing you make calls on" if they cannot think of the word "telephone."

- They may use more pat phrases that sound like regular social dialogue, which really cover up an inability to say more complex things. "Hello how are you? You look real good." May be repeated to each person they meet.

Helping the Person Communicate in the Middle Stage of Alzheimer's Disease

Never ask if the person in your care remembers the name of the person you have bumped into or the names of his six grandchildren. Avoid calling attention to memory problems and embarrassing him. If he says something that does not make perfect sense or behaves as if he remembers the person, don't correct him and say "No, we did not meet Jane in Cape Cod. She lives around the corner." It may be painful for you to witness his attempts at "normal" communication. Try to give the person with dementia an opportunity to enjoy social contact, but if he does not get the cue that it is time to stop talking, then you can say something about having to get some place soon.

Tip

Caregivers find it works best if you—

- remove distractions,

- always use short sentences, and

- use "yes" or "no" questions

As the illness progresses, it will have an impact on many aspects of daily life. Communication difficulties may appear more severe because the person may have hearing and vision loss as well as problems with judgment, impulse control, and planning. Thus, for example, a person in the middle stage may speak loudly on the bus, approach strangers as if they were long-lost relatives, and ask you why that lady over there is so fat.

Sometimes people with AD use salty language, which they never would have used before they became ill. Don't be offended. It is the disease speaking. Try to remind yourself that these embarrassing behaviors are symptoms of the illness and are not meant to humiliate you. If the person with AD understood what he was doing, he wouldn't do it.

Latter Part of Middle Stage

Toward the later part of the middle stage the person with dementia may speak very haltingly and you may not be able to make sense of what she is trying to say.

You may still be able to get the drift, however, and the feeling tone and you can respond to that as best you can. "That sounds important" may be a possible response and if the person is making an effort to express something, then it is important to her that you acknowledge it.

Family members should try to understand what the person with AD is trying to say, and to respond in a way he is likely to understand. When the person is among strangers, it may be necessary for family to explain to them what the ill person is saying and to convey what the others are saying to the ill person. You are acting as interpreter for both parties. You are more likely to be able to figure out what the person in your care is trying to say, since you know this person better than they do. You may have to repeat what was said to the person in your care in simpler terms. You may also want to gently help the person in your care to communicate with the other person. This is especially important when visiting the doctor, or when the person with AD is in the hospital (see *Health Care for the Person with Alzheimer's Disease*, p. 103, for more details).

NOTE Sometimes people with Alzheimer's disease whose first language was not English will no longer speak English and begin to speak only the language they learned earlier in life.

Late Stage

In the late stage, people with AD gradually lose their ability to speak. They may make sounds or moans or facial expressions that give you a clue as to how they are doing. If you think that the person is uncomfortable, try to change his position, offer a drink, play music, or do whatever you think may bring him some comfort. Watch the response to your efforts to see if you are on the right track. You can communicate your caring through gentle gestures and even singing an old favorite song.

The need for contact is still felt by the person in your care. People with AD want to be able to communicate. They may be very frustrated by their inability to do so verbally. Their tone of voice may tell you what their words cannot. Try to learn to read their body language. You too can express yourself to them with body language. They may be able to understand a hug or a pat on the arm when they don't understand affectionate words.

NOTE Recent research has found that the social part of the brain is the last to be impaired by AD. So it is important to provide opportunities for socializing, such as having a friend visit.

Communication Is Not Just Speaking

As much as 90% of our communication is non-verbal. When the person in your care can no longer communicate with words, you can communicate that you care about him by the *tone* of your voice. A hug speaks more clearly than words. Music and dancing can also be a kind of communication. People with Alzheimer's disease may be able to sing a song with you, even though they can no longer speak. Dancing together can communicate your affection for each other.

Tip

Regardless of the stage, speak gently to the person and maintain eye contact. Smile warmly and often. The person with Alzheimer's may not understand or respond, but will sense your feeling and react to that.

Don't Forget Hearing and Vision

Hearing Loss

Make sure the person has proper glasses or a hearing aid. A skilled audiologist can suggest listening devices for a confused person.

Communication will be more difficult if your relative has an uncorrected hearing loss. It is worth finding an audiologist who is able to test hearing of people with Alzheimer's disease, and trying to have a hearing aid fitted. While some older people are uncomfortable with hearing aids, others benefit greatly.

Poor Vision

Don't assume that the reason the person in your care doesn't recognize others is due to Alzheimer's disease without having his vision checked. If the person in your care does not see well, perhaps new glasses will help. In any case, rather than risking startling the person, it is best to say who you are as you approach.

> **NOTE** Remember, people with AD can get other illnesses, just like any other older adult. If the speech problem seems worse than it should be for the person's stage of AD, consult a physician. Loss of speech can also be caused by damage to the brain or lack of oxygen due to a stroke or brain injury.

RESOURCES>

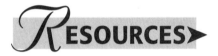

American Speech-Language-Hearing Association
10801 Rockville Pike
Rockville, MD 20852
(800) 638-8255
(301) 897-5700 (in Maryland)
www.asha.org
Provides free information on various communication disorders and makes referrals to audiologists and speech pathologists.

If you don't have home access to the Internet, ask your local library to help you locate any Web site.

Activities of Daily Living

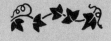

Activities of Daily Living

*H*elping with personal care is a major lifestyle change both for you and the person in your care. This is mainly true if you are caring for your parent, especially caring for a parent of the opposite sex. Even though it can be difficult to provide personal care to a parent, with time, most people adjust to the change in the relationship and are able to provide excellent care.

Alzheimer's disease gradually will get in the way of the person's ability to take care of activities of daily living— bathing, eating, toileting on her own. In the early stage, she will be able to do the activities without much help from you. But gradually you will need to provide more and more assistance so she can finish a task. In the late stage, the person will need total help.

It will be helpful if you think of these caregiving moments as opportunities to have a meaningful and pleasant shared experience, rather than as chores. If you approach the person with this attitude, it may be easier for him or her to accept your taking part in what used to be a private and ordinary part of the daily routine. As a caregiver, you also may feel less distressed by activities such as washing the person and touching private places if you think about them in that way. You may be saddened to see a person who once helped you coordinate your wardrobe stylishly now insisting she wants to wear the same thing every day.

In addition to dealing with these emotional aspects of providing care, as time goes by, it may be necessary for you to learn new skills, such as how to use adaptive devices such as shower chairs and hand-under-hand- assistance for helping the person in your care in the later stages. Training by an occupational or physical therapist will help you to be more competent and confident and will result in less stress for you and the person in your care.

Gentle Reminders

In the early stage of Alzheimer's disease you may simply need to *remind* the person to attend to his personal care needs. Some people with AD lose their former high standard of personal hygiene. This can be upsetting to the people around them. Sometimes this is because of his memory problems. For example, he may go into the bathroom to take a shower, forget why he is there, come back out, and when asked, say that he has showered. Remember, he is not lying, but saying what he thinks he is supposed to say or believes to be true. He may have forgotten whether or not he has showered and even get annoyed that you are questioning him.

As always, don't argue. You can suggest later that he shower. As with all personal care activities, try to follow the person's usual routine and to follow the same routine as much as possible from day to day. Most people are used to grooming in the early morning and then again late at night. If the person is able to do these tasks on his own, simply observe and make sure that the tasks are being done and not forgotten. These activities help provide a predictable structure for the day.

 Follow the same routine day to day. By knowing what to expect the person with dementia will be less likely to need to be told what to do and will have an internal sense of what is going to happen, giving him a sense of control.

How Much Care to Give

A person in the early stage, and even later, may enjoy going to the beauty parlor or barber shop as he or she always has. However, you may need to make the appointment for her, and then make sure she knows when it is time to go. Generally people in the early stage can manage most aspects of personal care on their own and you may only need to keep a friendly eye out for slipups.

In the middle stage your involvement in personal care will increase considerably even if the person does not have another medical condition that leaves him frail and in need of assistance. Otherwise healthy people in the middle stage are more confused, cannot plan their activities or make such previously simple choices as what to wear and the order in which clothing needs to be put on.

Bathing, dressing, eating, toileting, and mouth care are some of the activities of daily living that will require your assistance.

When helping a person with any activity, you will want to first give verbal instruction, than use visual gestures and finally, touch. It may be effective to combine a verbal cue with a gesture so that the person can get the information in more than one way. For instance, if you want the person to stand up, you can ask her to stand up, raise your hands up in a matching gesture and then if necessary touch her arm or leg to get her started. Only give as much help as is needed so that the person can remain as independent as possible. Offer encouraging words or a hug, to show your appreciation for their efforts.

To help the person in your care take part in caring for herself, use the hand-under-hand method shown on pp. 181–182. By guiding her hand you help her complete the motion and will possibly trigger a body memory of performing this task.

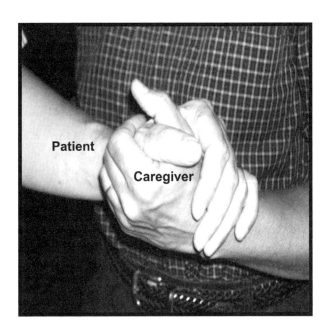

▶ *Hand-under-hand demonstration*

Patient

Caregiver

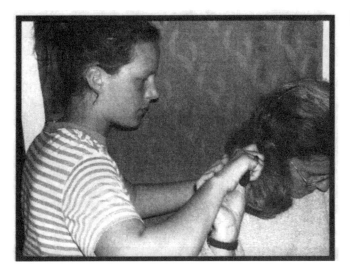

▶ *Hand-under-hand method of hair brushing*

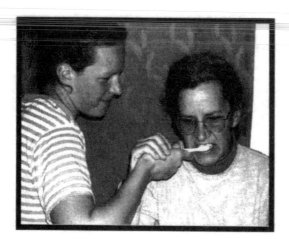

▶ *Hand-under-hand method of tooth brushing*

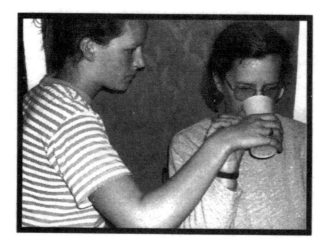

▶ *Hand-under-hand method of drinking from a cup*

Feelings About Providing Hands-On Care

At first you may feel overwhelmed as you review the list of tasks you will be performing when you care for a person with Alzheimer's disease. Some of these tasks will come to you automatically. Others you will need to learn how to do. It may feel uncomfortable at first to do for someone else what they formerly did for themselves. You will have to pay attention to details like drying between his toes.

In time you will develop a routine and confidence in your abilities. The person for whom you care may learn to cooperate with you as he becomes familiar with the routine. However, because the person has AD, there will be times when no matter what you do, things just don't work out as you planned. The person may get upset and be uncooperative. When this happens, try to step back, stay calm, and remember the ABCs of Alzheimer's care (see *Understanding Behavior in Alzheimer's Disease*, pp. 203–206). And don't forget—you don't have to do everything yourself, but it will be useful to know what to do and how to do it.

Eating

The ability of a person with Alzheimer's disease to make good food choices, to use utensils correctly, to chew and swallow his food, and to sit at the table changes over the course of the illness. As with other activities of daily living, people with Alzheimer's disease need more and more help as time passes.

At all stages mealtimes should be pleasant and can offer a social opportunity. They are a key time of the day. Allow plenty of time for each meal—a minimum of 30–45 minutes.

In the early stage you may not need to do anything special when preparing food, but may need to help with choosing a healthy diet. People with Alzheimer's can continue to eat without help for quite a while, but eventually they will begin to need help.

In the middle stage of AD, people need help choosing appropriate food. On their own, they may eat only food that is not healthy or is unsuitable for any medical conditions they may have. You don't want to become the food police and say "no" all the time, so keep items that are good for the person to eat readily available. When offering food, don't clutter the plate. When necessary, cut food into bite-size pieces. If the person wants to eat with his fingers, try not to be critical and offer finger food. Be aware that people in this stage may add too much salt or pepper to their food by mistake or put sugar rather than salt on a hamburger. It may be best to keep these condiments out of reach. In a restaurant you may have to remove them from the table.

In the middle stage of AD, people may be easily distracted while eating, so keep the environment calm. Turn off the television. Put music on the radio rather than a talk show. Sometimes, toward the end of the middle stage, people enjoy being fed even though they may still be able to feed themselves. They may not want this help all the time.

In the more severe stage you will have to pureé all the food and feed the person all the time. Be sure the person is sitting up straight enough so he will not choke. In the very end stage some people may want to drink from a bottle. This may be an effective way of feeding them.

NOTE People with dementia often seem to have a sweet tooth. Ice cream and other treats can be used to encourage them to finish either a meal or other activities. Place acceptable treats where they can be found easily and restricted items out of sight.

Eating Tips for the Middle Stage of AD

- Put only a few items on a plate and use a plain white plate. Serve the meal one course at a time to ensure the dessert does not come first, leaving no room or interest for healthier items.

- Be on the lookout for changes in eating behavior.

- Check temperature of food often. Name the food being offered.

- Provide finger foods if needed—a person may eat more independently and will have improved nutrition.

- When needed, cut foods into bite-size portions.

- Watch use of utensils. Don't put a knife on the table if the person can no longer use it properly.

- Watch for choking or problems swallowing. Consult a doctor or speech or occupational therapist if problems arise.

 Tip   Choose strong colors to help utensils stand out on the table.

Eating Tips for the Late Stage of AD

- In the late stage of Alzheimer's disease, you will need to cue the person to chew and swallow; give simple instructions—"open your mouth, move your tongue, now swallow, etc." If a person refuses to eat, don't force eating; provide a drink and return a little later and try again.

- Sometimes a rubber tipped spoon is better than metal.

- Feed at a steady pace, alternating food and drink.

When a person no longer wants to eat or is no longer able to swallow, the person who is the Health Care Proxy will have to decide whether to use a feeding tube or to allow the person's body to follow its natural course. When a person in an earlier stage of AD refuses to eat, consider depression, distress, physical problems, and other causes. A doctor's opinion may be needed.

People who pace a great deal use up a lot of calories and may need to have several snacks during the day to maintain their weight.

 Since people with AD are easily distracted, if necessary face his chair away from distractions. Soft music can help set a calm mood.

 Observing whether a person with Alzheimer's disease is able to make good food choices and the degree to which he is able to eat independently is a good way of tracking the progression of the illness.

Boosting Food Intake When the Appetite Is Poor

- Offer more food at the time of day when the person is most hungry or less tired.

- To increase the appeal of food for those with decreased taste and smell, provide strong flavors.

- Use milk or cream instead of water in soups and cooked cereal.

- Add fat by using butter, margarine, or olive oil on foods, unless this will worsen other medical conditions.

- Add nonfat dry-milk powder to foods like yogurt, mashed potatoes, gravy, and sauces.

- Don't stop the person from eating with his or her fingers if that is the only way to get the person to eat.

- Offer milk or fruit shakes.

- Offer puréed (finely ground) baby foods.

For more information on eating problems please refer to *The Comfort of Home™: A Complete Guide for Caregivers.*

Bathing

Bathing is often called the most challenging activity for both the person with dementia and the caregiver. What a shame that the idea of relaxing in a warm tub filled with bubbles rarely matches the typical caregiver–care receiver experience. Standing naked, afraid of falling, in a room that may be drafty, with water coming from all kinds of unexpected places may result in pain, fatigue, weakness, confusion, and anxiety for the person with Alzheimer's disease. These feelings may also exist before the bath and get worse because of the bath.

 Tip
If "bath" is a bad word, try saying, "Let's get ready for the day (or night as the case may be)."

To make bathing easier—

- **Let the person feel in control.**

  Does the person prefer showers, a tub bath, and at what time of day?

- **Create a safe atmosphere.**

  Put non-slip adhesives on the floor and bottom of tub, install grab bars to prevent falls, test the water temperature in advance

- **Use a bath bench.**

- **Respect the person's dignity.**

  Allow the person to keep a towel around him or her both in and out of the shower, if necessary

- **Don't worry about bathing.**

    It doesn't have to be done every day. Sponge baths can be used in between showers and baths.

- **Be gentle.**

    The person's skin may be sensitive. Avoid scrubbing. Pat dry, Use lotion.

- **Be flexible.**

    If the person does not want a shampoo use a wash cloth to soap and rinse the hair or a shampoo in a cap or no rinse shampoo can be substituted for a regular shampoo.

Talk with the person, tell him what you are going to do next, encourage him to wash areas that he can and watch that the flow of water so it is not too strong. These tips can contribute to making bathing a pleasant experience.

A person can also be washed in his room in bed, if showers or baths are not comfortable or feasible.

Bathing Tips:

- Water splashed on the face can be frightening for the person with Alzheimer's. It may be helpful to use a washcloth on the face.

- Running water can be scary. Face the person away from it. If you cannot wash the person's hair in the shower or bath, consider dry shampoo.

- Removing clothes can be frightening or painful and cause a feeling of loss. Don't rush.

- If you have to bathe someone and he refuses, consider waiting till after he takes a nap, and then use a sponge bath.

- Think of things that might relax the person—soft background music; make sure the bathroom is warm.

- Assistive items such as a shower with a hand-held nozzle, a shower chair in the stall, or a bath bench can be helpful if you know how to use them correctly.

- Use distractions if the person is nervous or uncomfortable to try to take his attention away from the water or what is scaring him.

- Have all necessary items at hand because you cannot leave the person alone to go get something.

Different techniques can be used depending on the needs of the person in your care. Here is a quick summary:

- *Bed bath*—this may be useful if the person must stay in bed. This is a also a good time to check for skin conditions such as bedsores or rashes. (For detailed instructions, see *The Comfort of Home™: A Complete Guide for Caregivers.*)

- *Basin bath*—if the person is in a chair or wheelchair, you can give a sponge bath at the sink.

- *Tub bath*—use if the person has good mobility and is strong enough to get into and out of the tub. Be careful—tubs can be dangerous if a person has problems with balance.

- *Shower*—make sure the floor is not slippery; let the person smell soap and feel a towel if he does not understand; make sure the room is warm.

In the advanced stage of dementia, bed or sponge baths may be the only choices you have.

For more detailed information and step-by-step instructions on all aspects of bathing, grooming, and oral care, see *The Comfort of Home™: A Complete Guide for Caregivers.*

 SKIN CARE
It is easier to prevent chapping than to heal it, so apply lotion often.

Dressing

In helping a person with Alzheimer's disease to select and put on clothing, be mindful of the choices he used to make, and try to honor that taste and style. For example, if an elderly man had worn a tie every day to work, but could no longer tie the knot and was frustrated if he could not put the tie on every day, a simple solution is to tie several in advance for him and let him slip the ties on and off. That may be easier for him to do and save you time. Sometimes a "clip on" tie will work also.

NOTE Clean out closets and drawers so that out of season or difficult to clean clothes will not be temptingly in view.

Most people have favorite colors, textures, and types of clothing—and people with dementia often want to wear the same outfit all the time. If you get duplicates of the items the person always wants to wear, he can still be comfortable when clothes are being washed and you will avoid arguments and explanations.

Tip If the person wants to wear something you don't like, try to accept his choice, unless it is totally inappropriate.

Lay out clothing in the order in which it should be put on. This will provide a cue to those who are unsure what to put on next, and will generally make the process run more smoothly when you have to assist. You will also not need to leave the person to go find a missing piece.

- Use clothes that are easy to put on.

- Store all like clothes together.

- Use shoes that slip on or fasten with Velcro®.

- Use socks rather than pantyhose.

- Use pants and skirts with elastic waistbands.

- Use bras with front openers.

- Avoid clothes that have to be put on over the head.

- Replace buttons with Velcro closures.

Sometimes, people with Alzheimer's disease will undress at inappropriate times. If it is because he is fidgeting and unintentionally opening buttons, consider sweaters without buttons, or a one-piece jump suit. Sometimes, wearing an apron will be a distraction. If things are sewn onto the apron, that will give the person something to touch and feel with his hands, distracting him from trying to remove a shirt or pants.

It may be best to have a frail person or someone with poor balance or a disability sit down when you help dress him, unless of course he is bed bound. If the person has a "weak" side, dress it first.

NOTE For a person who is confined to bed, be sure to smooth out all wrinkles in the clothes and bedding to prevent pressure sores.

Toileting

Incontinence usually begins in the late part of the middle stage of AD. It is a symptom of Alzheimer's disease that caregivers fear they will not be able to handle. Many learn to take it in stride and find that it is not the "deal breaker" they expected it to be. Knowing how to use the proper products will help you with the discomfort you may feel.

Confusion about how to find the bathroom, inability to get there on time, or a urinary tract infection may be the cause of the problem. Be sure to ask the doctor if there could be a physical cause of the problem, rather than the progression of AD.

 Tip   A regular toileting schedule and reading the signals when the person needs to go to the toilet may help the person to continue to use the toilet for a longer time. However, you will probably need to use protection for the bed since the person may sleep through the need to go.

Other suggestions for reducing the problems of incontinence:

- Always be calm and understanding when accidents occur.

- Wear gloves. This prevents the spread of disease; wash hands before and after assistance.

- If the person cannot use the toilet and cannot learn to use a urinal, commode, or in-bed toileting, incontinence products will be necessary. If the person can move around on his own, do not encourage bed toileting.

- Watch for signs of urinary tract infection (blood in urine, cloudy urine with sediment, etc.).

- Because he may not recognize the need to use the toilet, "suggestions" to go to the bathroom can be very helpful—just a simple reminder after a meal, for example, or early in the morning, or before bedtime.

- If the person is in the early stage of AD, leave a bathroom light on at night so a person can find the bathroom easily. If it is in another room, make sure the "pathway" is marked. Marking a path can be done with something simple, such as reflecting tape. A person with middle-stage AD cannot toilet himself independently. Some caregivers will wake the person at night to take him to the bathroom, while others prefer to use incontinence products.

 You may need to try different incontinence products before you find the one that works best for the person in your care. Some companies are willing to send sample packages to let you experiment with different styles, shapes, and closures.

Using a Commode

A portable commode is helpful for a person with limited mobility. The portable commode (with the pail removed) can be used over the toilet seat and as a shower seat.

Using the Bathroom Toilet

If the mobile person is missing the toilet, get a toilet seat in a color that is different from the floor color. This may help him see the toilet better. If the person with AD fails to remember to wipe himself or wash his hands, you will have to prompt him to do it, help him to do it, or do it for him.

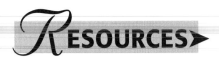

Meeting Life's Challenges
9042 Aspen Grove Lane
Madison, WI 53717
Fax (608) 824-0403
www.meetinglifeschallenges.com
E-mail: help@meetinglifeschallenges.com
Offers a guide called Dressing Tips and Clothing Resources for Making Life Easier, *by Shelley P. Schwarz, a guide to dressing for people with disabilities plus more than 100 resources for custom clothing.*

The Alzheimer's Store
(800) 752-33238
www.alzstore.com
Carries unique products and information for caregivers of people with AD. Products are designed to make living with AD as easy as possible.

Connections Newsletter vol. 14, issue 3 (2006) "Encouraging Eating: Advice for At-Home Dementia Caregivers"
http://www.nia.nih.gov/Alzheimers/Research/
Information

Activities of Daily Living—An ADL Guide for Alzheimer's Care by Kathy Laurenhue.
Wiser Now, Inc.
Bradenton, FL 34202
(800) 999-0795
Email: Kathy@wisernow.com

If you don't have home access to the Internet, ask your local library to help you locate any Web site.

Understanding Behavior in Alzheimer's Disease

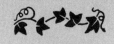

Understanding Behavior in Alzheimer's Disease

*I*t may be that for years, even before you thought of seeking an explanation for the changes in the person in your care, deterioration in his brain was causing him to behave in ways that made you think he was "not himself." Changes in mood and interests, and the inability to find his way occasionally were perhaps chalked up to senior moments, not paying attention, and maybe even to poor sleep habits. But looking back on these incidents, now that he has been diagnosed with Alzheimer's disease, you know that many of these changes in behavior were early signs of the illness.

Early-Stage Behaviors—Decisions, Decisions

In the early stage of the illness, it is common for caregivers (who may not yet even call themselves caregivers), to wonder how much the person can still do on his own, and when they should step in and be protective.

These are some of the questions to ask yourself. Is it safe for the person to—

- continue driving? (see *Special Occasions and Challenges*, p. 239)

- continue to work?

- take medications on his own?

- travel on his own?

- make financial decisions that he has been making until now?

You will continually have to evaluate the benefits and risks for the person in your care and the people around him. Is the risk that something bad will happen worth taking in order to prolong his independence? On the one hand, he may very much want to continue to drive, but if he has an accident because he cannot drive safely, someone may get hurt or killed. That is a too big a risk, regardless of the reward. On the other hand, if the person wants to dress himself and cannot select matching clothes, there is no risk, and a lot to gain by letting him dress himself.

Although you cannot alter the effects of the disease, you can learn the best ways to respond to the behaviors that are caused by the disease.

Remember: The person with Alzheimer's disease is always doing the best he can.

Balancing Safety and Risk

How can you decide what is safe versus what is not? The doctor who conducted the diagnostic evaluation can help you to answer this question. Independent driving tests can be arranged. Your own experience and observations of the person can help you to decide what to do. Your friends and family may have noticed something you did not. If you or other people feel anxious because of unsafe driving, you cannot ignore the problem. Attending meetings at the Alzheimer's Association and reading information in books and on the Internet will give you more information.

Your decisions will be easier to carry out if the person with dementia is aware of the diagnosis and understands that he will not be able to do things he did in the past.

However, often the person denies the changes and resists your efforts to limit his activities. In this case, other family members, friends, or neighbors may be able to help you work around the problem. They may offer to drive you and him where you need to go or perform other activities without mentioning that it is because the person is no longer able to do them.

It is useless to try to convince the person of the need to give up valued activities. **Remember: Arguing or insisting never helps.** The person will only resist you more strongly.

Decision-Making Ability

It is important to keep in mind that the person in the early stage of Alzheimer's can continue to do many of the things he has always done. However, one important ability that is often lost early is making decisions, even such seemingly simple ones as what to order in a restaurant.

Repetition

People in the early stage of AD frequently ask the same question over and over because they quickly forget both that they have asked and what was answered. Questions tend to be about upcoming events, such as going to the doctor. They are aware that something is going to happen, but don't remember what. This makes them anxious. Generally, the best response is to simply repeat the answer to the question as if it had never been asked before and guide the person to another activity.

Lack of Initiative

The person in your care may also put off making dates with friends or calling to make an appointment with the doctor. This is called *lack of initiative*. It may be the person's way of avoiding difficult or uncomfortable situations or it may be a symptom of changes in the brain. Whatever the cause, try *not* to remind the person about what he is not doing. Instead focus on the strengths that remain. Continue to enjoy as many of the activities you used to do together as you can, such as listening to music or taking walks.

Middle-Stage Behaviors—Time for More Hands-On Care

As the illness progress to the middle stage there will no longer be any doubt that the person has an illness. As time goes on, you will need to learn how to help the person with AD with what are called "activities of daily living," which include choosing the right clothes, maintaining good hygiene, taking medications, and eating the right foods (📖 see *Activities of Daily Living*, p. 177). You should also think about organizing the day so she is not rushed or bored. Plan several activities. It is important that she get some stimulation, but not so much that she becomes overwhelmed (📖 see *Setting Up a Plan for Day-to-Day Activities*, p. 139).

During the middle stage of the illness you will have to take a more hands-on approach to care because the person needs more supervision and help with activities of daily living. This is also the stage when what are often called "difficult behaviors" generally occur, although some may have already begun. When care is provided in a sympathetic and skillful way, these behaviors may not occur, or may not be as severe or burdensome.

> **Tip**
>
> Remember the person's typical habits, likes, and dislikes. Give him the right to say "no" when he doesn't feel like taking a bath or doing something else you ask him to do. If possible, try again later, rather than forcing the issue just because it is a convenient time for you. And sometimes you may need to just let the activity go. *Just let it go.*

NOTE Remember, these behaviors are caused by both the effects of the illness on the brain, which **is losing cells, and is congested with plaques and tangles,** and the way you and others interact with and care for the person. The person with AD cannot control his behavior, but *you* can control *yours.* You'll feel better when you do.

Medications

In some situations, when changes in the environment and the way care is provided have not worked, certain medications may help the person to be more cooperative and comfortable. Medications have side effects and don't work for every person, so be prepared to work with your doctor to find the best one (see *Health Care for the Person with Alzheimer's Disease,* p. 108).

How to Deal with Common Difficult Behaviors

In your caregiving you will find some behaviors more difficult to deal with than others. You will need to learn skillful ways of coping both with the behavior *and* how to keep yourself from caregiver burnout (see *How To Avoid Caregiver Burnout*, p. 152).

Your reaction depends on how you interpret the behavior. If you can think of these behaviors as the person with Alzheimer's way of communicating what she needs and feels or what is upsetting her, you may have an easier time responding calmly.

If you believe that she is not trying hard enough or is being spiteful, you will probably react in an angry way that will only make the situation worse for both of you.

Here are some practical everyday things to consider when a person is behaving in a way that is making life difficult for both of you.

Check if the person in your care may be—

- feeling ill
- in pain
- having a reaction to a medication
- overtired
- not able to understand what you want her to do
- just not in the mood for what you have in mind
- bored or overstimulated
- having a bad day—symptoms often vary from day to day

Check if you are—

- trying to make her do something at a different time of day
- expecting too much for her skills
- rushing her
- giving too many directions at once
- speaking in an angry or bossy way
- stressed out

Checklist Tips on How to Use a Positive Approach

✓ **Come toward the person from the front** so he can see you coming. Don't come from behind him, which may surprise or frighten him. Keep in mind that as they age, people have a narrower field of vision, which means they may not see people or objects that are not right in front of them.

✓ **Speak and move slowly but not so slowly the person forgets the beginning of the sentence.** People with Alzheimer's disease take more time to process information. (What feels slow to you may seem fast to him.)

✓ **Stand to the side.** When you are near the person who is sitting down, stand to the side. Standing right in front and towering over the person may seem confrontational.

✓ **Bend to his level.** If the person is sitting, especially in a wheelchair, bend down so you are at his level. You don't want to be towering over a person.

✓ **Identify yourself.** Use his name and identify yourself, even if you are sure he knows you. At that moment, he may not remember who you are. You could say something like, "Hello George darling. It's me, Alice, your wife."

✓ **Tell him what you want him to do in as few words as possible.** (For further discussion of the best ways to communicate with a person who has Alzheimer's disease, see *Understanding and Improving Communication,* p. 168).

Used with permission from Positive Physical Approach developed by Teepa Snow, MS, ORT/L FAOTA, 2000, revised for Eastern North Carolina Alzheimer's Association Caregiver Training Programs, 2002, revised 2006.

Check the environment. Is it comfortable?

- Is the room too noisy, smelly, crowded, unfamiliar?
- Is the room too hot or too cold?
- Does the room look scary? For example, bathrooms with all kinds of appliances that no longer seem familiar to her can be frightening.
- Was there a recent change in residence or of caregiver?

Ask yourself if the task *must* be done. When a person resists your care, you will also want to ask yourself—

- Is it essential that I do this now?
- Is it essential that I do this at all?
- What is the person's behavior telling me?

Tip

It is important to think about the person's behavior from his perspective and then to ask yourself what would be the best way to help. Are you willing to change your expectations and approach? *Remember, the person with Alzheimer's has great difficulty making decisions. He cannot* decide *to change. Can you?*

The ABC Way to Understand Alzheimer's Behavior

A person with Alzheimer's disease may sometimes act in ways that are upsetting or seem aggressive. He or she may hit, scratch, or fight with the caregiver. This does not always happen. But if it does, it is likely to be when the person is in the middle stage of Alzheimer's disease. This stage can last for up to four years.

These actions can be upsetting and are often hard for caregivers to manage. It helps to have a plan. One that many people find easy to remember is called ABC. Here is what this means:

A means Antecedent. This refers to events that happen just before an upsetting action.

B is the Behavior. This means any upsetting or aggressive action done by the person who has Alzheimer's disease.

C refers to the Consequence. This includes events that happen after the behavior. Sometimes, these events can make the situation worse.

Here is a story about people we are calling Mary and Robert Jones. In this story, Mary is the caregiver for her husband, Robert, who has Alzheimer's disease. As you will see, in this story many things go wrong.

A. The Antecedent. What happened before the behavior?

Mary slept too late and now is in a hurry. She wants her husband Robert to quickly get out of bed, take a shower, eat, and get dressed before a driver arrives to take them to his doctor's appointment. Because of her late start, Mary yanks off the bed covers and yells at Robert to get up. He does not understand the words but reacts to her tone of voice. Mary gets angry when he pulls the bed covers back up. "So that's the way it will be. I'm in charge here," she yells.

Mary then drags Robert out of bed and rushes to get him dressed. Now he must balance on one leg rather than sit down to pull up his pants. This is not their usual routine when Mary takes her time helping Robert get ready for the day.

B. The Behavior.

Robert loses his balance because Mary is rushing him so much. He grabs her arm for support and does not let go. When she yells, he grabs even tighter. Robert is now digging his nails into Mary's arm.

C. The Consequence. The events that followed the behavior.

Mary loses control and smacks Robert in the face (something she had never done before). He hits her back. Mary thinks he is fighting, though it may be that he is just afraid and doing to her what she did to him.

One problem leads to others and Mary now worries that Robert will hurt her again. She questions whether she can care for him at home and wonders whether Robert must go to a nursing home.

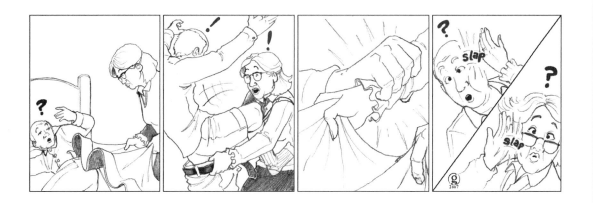

Now let's look again at this story using the ABC way. Mary can see that the problems started when she rushed around and did not think of how Robert would react. She now knows she must avoid these types of situations.

- Mary learned that because Robert has Alzheimer's disease, he cannot be rushed. While she should not feel guilty, she should realize how her actions made this worse.

- If Mary is ever late again, she will call the doctor's office and ask if they can make a new appointment or come in later in the day. This is better than expecting Robert to change his behavior.

- Mary will make a list of what happened just before Robert's upsetting behavior. She will look for *causes* of what went wrong and figure out ways to avoid them.

- Mary will also think about her own actions and what did or did not work well.

- Mary will use the ABC way to help Robert to be more cooperative in the future. This is a way to understand what happened, and figure out ways to better manage in the future.

Behaviors Caregivers Find Especially Difficult

There are some behaviors that caregivers find especially difficult. Not all people with Alzheimer's disease have these behaviors. However, it is likely that the person in your care will have one or more of these problems during the middle stage of Alzheimer's disease. It is important to try to understand why the person may be behaving in ways you find difficult, and learn how to avoid making them worse.

Agitation

The term "agitation" covers a group of different, but related, behaviors. Very mild agitation may seem like a personality change in which a person acts in ways that are uncharacteristic or inappropriate for him or her, such as being very stubborn, worried, or nervous. More severe agitation can be disruptive or even dangerous. Agitated behavior can start in the early stage and grows worse in the middle stage of the illness.

An agitated person may seem to be uneasy and becomes irritable, anxious, and moody. The person may be unable to sleep, pace constantly, move around restlessly, checking on doors, tearing paper, or even cursing or using threatening language.

If a person with dementia has recently become agitated for the first time or acts unlike her usual self, the first thing to look for is a medical or physical problem.

People with dementia are very sensitive to the environment they live in. They are less able to handle changes, uncertainty, and other situations that they could manage when they were well. Being in a strange place may cause agitation. Even a positive event, such as a wedding, can feel overwhelming to a person with Alzheimer's disease and can lead to agitation. If the person in your care has had a recent hospitalization or other major life change, expect to see some agitation or other expression of stress. It is important to evaluate your relative's environment to see if it is causing problems that may be adding to the agitation (📖 see *Preparing the Home*, p. 22).

 Try not to get agitated yourself when the person with AD does. Take a few breaths, stay calm, don't raise your voice, or take personally anything the person says (📖 *see How to Avoid Caregiver Burnout*, p. 151).

Don't forget that what used to bother the person in your care probably still will. While agitation may be a symptom of the illness, remember that you may have done something to offend the person that would have been distressing even before he became ill with Alzheimer's. If you realize you did something that upset him, apologize.

> **NOTE** A person with AD may not understand the words, but he ***will understand the tone of your voice.*** Keep your compassion and humanity and that of the person in your care in mind at all times, and you will provide better care.

Physically Aggressive Behavior

At some point in the course of the disease, people with Alzheimer's may become physically aggressive, although this does not occur as often as people think. They may sometimes throw things, hit, kick, bite, or pinch the caregiver or others they come into contact with. They may not know why they are doing this, and they may not even realize that they are doing it. These displays of behavior can be very frightening. Try to remember that these behaviors are probably an indication that the person with AD is very upset about something.

When it looks like he is getting upset, and may seem to be spoiling for a fight, perhaps using threatening language, you may feel frightened and tempted to fight back. Try to stay calm, use a reassuring tone, and distract the person.

Tip Usually, the person with Alzheimer's disease will calm down in a few minutes if you do not bother him.

Steps to Avoid Injury

Don't try to restrain the person. This could cause serious injury to both of you.

1. Get out of striking distance. Step away so that he cannot reach you.

2. Call for help if you need it. You can call a friend, family member, or neighbor to help you get the person

calmed down. If you have to, you can also call 911 or your local emergency number.

3. Try to avoid creating a situation in which the person with AD will feel threatened because this will only make him more upset. When things have calmed down figure out what has set the person off using the ABC method on p. 203.

What seems like violent behavior may be the way this person is responding to changes in his brain or to events that he doesn't understand, and interprets as dangerous in some way. These might be an unfamiliar person entering the room, attempts to take something away from him, fear of being hurt, an exaggerated response to something happening suddenly, not knowing how to express anger appropriately, or just an effort to avoid complying with a demand.

It is easy to forget that what you think is a very natural way to behave may seem frightening or threatening to a confused person with dementia. So remember the steps in the positive approach described on page 203, and you may avoid these distressing events.

Sleep Disturbances in Alzheimer's Disease

Changes in the brain can alter the sleep patterns of people with dementia. The body clock may not function as well as it did before. Like anyone who has problems falling asleep or staying asleep, having a daily schedule with enough activity and periods of rest, avoiding caffeine in the later part of the day, and sticking to a regular time for 1going to bed may help. Sleep medications should be used only as a last resort. Discuss them with the doctor before using them.

Sometimes the person with Alzheimer's disease will want to sleep in the clothes he has worn during the day. He may prefer to sleep in a comfortable chair in the living room instead of in bed. If there is no harm in going along with these behaviors, do not make an issue about them. However, be sure that the house is securely locked so if the person wakes up and wants to go outside during the night while others are sleeping, he cannot do so.

Sundowning

People with Alzheimer's disease may become more confused, restless, or insecure late in the afternoon or early evening, when the sun is going down. It can be worse after a move or a change in their routine. They may become suspicious or see and hear things that are not there. No one is sure what causes sundowning. Here are some other possible causes—

• an upset in the "internal body clock," causing a biological mix-up between day and night

• less need for sleep, which is common among older adults

• the person can't see well in dim light and becomes confused

• the person gets tired at the end of the day and is less able to cope with stress

• the person is involved in activities all day long and grows restless if there's nothing to do in the late afternoon or evening

• the caregiver communicates fatigue and stress to the person and he becomes anxious

Tips to Make Sundowning Behaviors Less Likely

• If fatigue is making the sundowning worse, an early afternoon rest might help.

• Keep the person active in the morning and encourage a rest after lunch.

• Early-evening activities that are familiar from an earlier time in the person's life may be helpful, such as "paper work" for a former secretary or planting seeds for a gardener.

- Closing the curtains, having a predinner nonalcoholic drink, or assisting with preparing dinner or setting the table may be helpful.

- Don't physically restrain the person. Let her pace where she is safe. A walk outdoors can help reduce restlessness.

- Some people are comforted by soft toy animals, pets, hearing familiar tunes, or an opportunity to follow a favorite pastime.

- Consider the effect of bright lights and noise from television and radios. Are these adding to the confusion and restlessness?

- Try not to arrange baths or showers for the late afternoon if these are upsetting activities. The exception may be the person who is calmed by a hot bath before bed.

- Nightlights or a radio playing softly may help the person sleep.

- Some people find warm milk, a back rub, or music calming.

- Some may need medication. This will need to be discussed with the doctor.

- Make sure you get plenty of rest yourself as caregiver.

(Tips from Gwyther, L. P. (1985). *Care of Alzheimer's Patients: A Manual for Nursing Home Staff.*)

Sexual Behavior

Sometimes people with dementia touch or expose their genitals in public, or try to touch others in ways that are considered inappropriate. You may feel embarrassed or even disgusted but try not to get judgemental.

> **Tip**
>
> Ask yourself what the behavior is telling you. It may be as simple as clothing being too tight or wet, or he needs to use the bathroom. It may be that he is trying to express affection, or longing for physical contact and sexual expression.

If you are his spouse or partner, you may also be missing the hugs, kisses, and sex that used to be a part of your relationship, and you may be able to respond in a way that makes both of you happier. Maybe some hugs and tender touch can meet both your needs. If you are not the spouse or partner, or his attempts bother you, try to divert his attention. He is likely to quickly forget the attempt.

Wandering

One of the most troubling aspects of Alzheimer's is the person's tendency to wander away from home.

Why People with Alzheimer's Wander

There is no way to predict who will wander or when it might happen. However, some of the reasons for wandering are:

- pain
- boredom
- side effects of medication
- a noisy or stressful environment
- confusion about time
- an attempt to meet basic needs (finding the toilet)
- restlessness
- being in an unfamiliar environment

- trying to meet former obligations (to job, home, friends, family)

Wandering may also be a natural release for boredom or agitation. If this is the reason, wandering within a safe, confined space may be encouraged. Some recent research suggests that more socially oriented people will wander in an effort to make contact with others. When faced with episodes of wandering, try to find their cause.

What Happens When People with AD Wander

- Of those with Alzheimer's or a related dementia, 59% will get lost, usually while doing normal activities.

- Of those not located within 24 hours of the last time seen, 46% may die, usually succumbing to cold and thirst.

- Individuals with Alzheimer's usually do not cry out for help or respond to shouts; they leave few physical clues.

- They usually travel less than one-tenth of a mile.

- They may try to travel to a former residence, work place, or city.

- They are usually found a short distance from a road or an open field; 63% are found in a creek or drainage area or caught in briars or bushes.

- Most wandering incidents occur during normal daily activities (while trying to locate a restroom, gift shop, recreation room, etc.).

How to Reduce the Chance of Wandering

You cannot always prevent wandering, but you can do many things to reduce the chances that it will happen.

- Provide opportunities for exercise, particularly when the person is waiting for a meal or an activity. Exercise might include singing, rhythmic movements, walking at an indoor mall track, or dancing.

- Develop areas indoors and outdoors where the person can explore and wander independently.

- Clearly label bathrooms, living rooms, and bedrooms with large letters or pictures.

- Try a yellow strip of plastic, symbolizing caution, that is attached with Velcro® across doors to prevent wanderers from entering or leaving the room.

- Camouflage doors by painting exit doors the same color as the walls.

- Cover doors with curtains.

- Install electronic alarms or chimes on windows and doors.

- Place a large stop sign or do not enter sign on doors.

- Place a full-length mirror on doors to the outside. Some people will turn around when they see the image, not recognizing themselves. (📖 See *Preparing the Home,* p. 44.)

- Monitor medications and medication changes, especially anti-depressants or anti-anxiety drugs as they may be making the person agitated and increasing the risk of wandering.

- Determine whether wandering is related to previous lifestyles. Find out how the person coped with change and stress and learn about patterns of physical exercise and lifetime habits, both at home and at work. (Did the person always react to an argument by going out and walking for an hour? Did he always jog in the afternoon?)

- Have a plan of action if wandering occurs.

- Keep a photo on hand to give the police if an incident occurs.

- Keep unwashed clothing. Wipe the person's face or arm with clean cotton balls that can be stored in individual Ziploc bags in the freezer. (Tracking dogs can use them to pick up a scent.)

Alzheimer's Association Safe Return® Program

It's common for a person with Alzheimer's or a related dementia to wander and become lost. Many do so repeatedly. This can be dangerous, even life threatening. The stress can weigh heavily on family and caregivers. Since 1993, the Alzheimer's Association Safe Return® program has helped reunite more than 13,000 people with their families and caregivers.

An authorized caregiver or family member can enroll a person with dementia into the Alzheimer's Association's Safe Return® program by submitting a completed enrollment form with a $40 enrollment fee. For an additional $15 matching caregiver jewelry is available, which will alert others to look after the person with dementia should the caregiver become disabled. After one year, there is a $20 annual program administration fee that helps Safe Return respond to the more than 6,000 calls for help each year. Having the identifying information and a picture stored in a national database will increase the chances of finding someone should they wander or become lost.

Tip   Ask if the fee can be waived, or if there is a free enrollment plan available.

> **NOTE** Update enrollment information regularly as this can be of great value to the police. The more current information you provide, the better the chances of finding the individual. To report someone missing or found call the Safe Return Hotline at (800) 572-1122. Representatives are available to help 24 hours a day, everyday. If the enrollee moves or goes on vacation, call (888) 572-8566 to update information as soon as possible.

Encouraging Use of Safe Return ID Products

- Wrap the jewelry in a box and present it as a gift.

- Have a grandchild present the jewelry. (The person may appreciate the gesture and wear the jewelry.)

- If the person has a medical appointment soon after receiving the jewelry, ask the doctor to place it on the person during the appointment. It may be better received from the doctor.

- Place the bracelet on the individual's dominant hand. This will make it more difficult to undo the clasp.

- Keep the bracelet comfortable—neither too tight nor too loose. A bracelet that is too loose may be easy to remove.

- If a person is comfortable wearing a watch or other jewelry on only one wrist, place the bracelet on the same wrist.

- Find creative places for the individual to wear the jewelry. Attach it to a belt loop or purse handle, or place it on the shoe laces.

- Wear Safe Return caregiver's jewelry yourself.

- If the person is not comfortable wearing a bracelet, an ID necklace is available.

- For someone who will not wear the bracelet or necklace, use the ID clothing labels, wallet cards, and key chain that are included with the enrollment packet.

If the Person Is Missing

- Search the immediate area where the person was last seen; most people are found within a half-mile of where they were last seen.

- Call the police. Tell them that the person is memory impaired and at risk. Let them know it is urgent to locate him or her quickly.

- Inform the police of the special danger areas in your neighborhood.

- Provide them with a photo.

- Describe what the person was last wearing in as much detail as possible.

- Inform the police about special medical conditions and medications.

- Call Safe Return, (800) 572-1122, to report the person missing. Have the enrollee's ID number available.

- Call your family, friends or neighbors and ask them to continue the search.

- Stay where you are, stay by the phone, keep phone lines open, and stay calm.

- Call hospital emergency rooms. (Someone may have taken the person there.)

- Call transit systems to alert drivers.

- Call your local chapter of the Alzheimer's Association.

When the missing person is found, call the police and the Safe Return program (1-800-572-1122) to inform them.

Information about the Safe Return Program is adapted with permission from the Alzheimer's Association © 2006.

People with Alzheimer's disease may see, hear, smell, taste, or feel things that are not really there. The most common hallucinations are those that involve sight or hearing. Some people with Alzheimer's disease develop strange ideas about what is actually happening and may come to believe that other people want to harm them. This kind of belief is called a *delusion*.

These symptoms are usually thought of as being caused by mental illness, but they are actually fairly common in Alzheimer's disease, especially in the middle stage, although they can occur at other stages. There may be many causes mostly having to do with the parts of the brain affected by the disease. In any case, it is important not to be frightened by what are irrational thoughts and experiences and to know how to respond to them.

It is essential that you do not tell the person who is seeing or hearing things that you know what he sees is not real because the things are real to the person. Reassure the person that you will keep him safe and try to *understand the emotion behind the hallucination or delusion*. This may be enough to enable the person to let go of these concerns, at least for the moment. If the hallucination is pleasant and the person is planning a birthday party, try to connect to her by joining in the fantasy. You do not need to say that you see or hear the same things but you can accept that the person does.

People with Alzheimer's disease may also become suspicious and may accuse someone of stealing from them when they cannot find something. When the person with dementia does not remember where he put something, the idea that it has been taken by someone may appear to be a reasonable explanation for its being missing. Tell him you will help him look for it, and try not to mention the fact that he is the one who misplaced it. He may feel relieved when the object is found.

Paranoia in people with Alzheimer's disease appears as unrealistic beliefs, usually of someone seeking to do them harm. They may hoard or hide things because they believe someone is trying to take their possessions. These symptoms can be very distressing both for the person with AD and for you. Remember, what the person is experiencing is very real to him. It is best not to argue or disagree. Try not to take it personally. In this situation it is best to offer to help the person to find the missing item. It will not be helpful to try to convince him that his explanation is wrong or based on his poor memory.

When these behaviors do not respond to supportive caregiving techniques it may be necessary to consider medication, especially if the person is very upset or puts himself or others in danger because of his symptoms. These symptoms are sometimes caused by depression, which often accompanies Alzheimer's disease. Consult with your physician, who may recommend an antidepressant medication. Other medications, called anti-psychotics, are frequently prescribed. They should be used with caution and sensitivity.

"Resistance" to Care

In the later part of the middle stage of Alzheimer's disease, when a person for whom you care seems to be refusing to cooperate with the activities of daily living such as dressing or bathing, you may think he is resisting care. In fact any time a person with Alzheimer's says "no" he may be labelled uncooperative.

People with Alzheimer's disease may get upset when somebody touches them. You may be trying to do something to help him, but he doesn't understand what's going on. He may be feeling uncomfortable, powerless, frightened, tired, in pain, or confused. He cannot say how he wants to be treated.

Resistance has many components. Try to put yourself in the shoes of the person with Alzheimer's disease and you may be able to avoid causing resistance. You may be able to change your approach to reduce these responses and actually be able to help the person to cooperate with you. See *Activities of Daily Living*, p. 177, and Tips on How to Use a Positive Approach (p. 202) for information on avoiding the battle of the bath and other daily activities.

Think about what it would feel like to constantly be told to do something you may not feel like doing or cannot understand what is expected of you.

In order to provide good care you need to know how to respond to all the different ways in which the illness affects the person with dementia. This means that in many cases the person shows you with actions what can no longer be communicated in words. So behaviors are more than behaviors. They are messages about ideas, feelings, and needs the person is telling you about in the best way he or she can.

The best thing you as caregiver can do is always ask yourself "What is he trying to say by doing this?"

After the Middle Stage

As the illness progresses to the late stage, the behaviors described in this chapter will no longer occur. The person will gradually lose the ability to walk, and be confined to a wheelchair and eventually to bed.

Your care will be focused on activities of daily living with which the person will need full assistance. The person may make sounds that disturb you, such as moaning and groaning. These behaviors may be an effort to communicate or may be the result of the neurological condition itself. The late stage will present new caregiving challenges, but the stress of dealing with the earlier behaviors will be behind you. (See *The Comfort of Home™: A Complete Guide for Caregivers*, 3rd ed., for detailed information on how to care for a person confined to bed.)

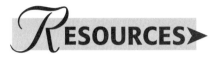

RESOURCES➤

Alzheimer's Association
225 North Michigan Avenue
Chicago, IL 60601
(312) 335-8700
(800) 272-3900
TDD (312) 335-8882
http://www.alz.org
Provides free literature and can refer you to your nearest local chapter that assists caregivers and family members.

Alzheimer's Association Safe Return® Program
P.O. Box A3687
Chicago, IL 60690-3687
For enrollment information and other safety services, call Safe Return at (888) 572-8566. For assistance with a wandering incident, call (800) 572-1122.

Alzheimer's Disease Education and Referral Center
P.O. Box 8250
Silver Spring, MD 20907
(800) 438-4380
Fax (301) 495-3334
http://www.alzheimers.org/adear
Sponsored by the National Institute on Aging, this organization provides information and publications on Alzheimer's disease to caregivers and the public.

American Health Assistance Foundation
15825 Shady Grove Road
Suite 140
Rockville, MD 20850
(800) 437-AHAF (2423)
http://www.ahaf.org
Provides a variety of written material on Alzheimer's disease.

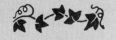

Moving, Transfers, and Falls

Moving, Transfers, and Falls

Body Mechanics for the Caregiver

Body mechanics involves standing and moving one's body to prevent injury, avoid fatigue, and make the best use of strength. When you learn how to control and balance your own body, you can safely control and move another person. Back injuries to caregivers are common, so when doing any lifting be sure to use proper body mechanics.

General Rules

- Never lift more than you can comfortably handle.

- Create a base of support by standing with your feet 8 to 12″ (shoulder width) apart with one foot a half step ahead of the other.

Proper foot position. ▶

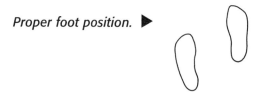

- DO NOT let your back do the heavy work—USE YOUR LEGS. (The back muscles are not your strongest muscles.)

- If the bed is low, put one foot on a footstool. This relieves pressure on your lower back.

- Consider using a support belt for your back.

Preventing Back and Neck Injuries

To prevent injuries to yourself, get plenty of rest and maintain:

- good nutrition
- physical fitness
- good body mechanics
- a program for managing stress

Common Treatments for Caregiver Back Pain

If you *do* experience back pain:

- Apply a cold ice pack to the injured area for 10 minutes every hour (you can use a bag of frozen vegetables).
- Get short rest periods in a comfortable position.
- Stand with your feet shoulder width apart. With hands on hips, bend backwards. Do 3 to 5 repetitions several times a day.
- Take short, frequent walks on a level surface.
- Avoid sitting for long periods. Sitting is one of the worst healing positions.

As the caregiver, you should seek training from a physical therapist to provide this type of care to reduce the risk of injury to yourself or the person in your care. The therapist will correct any mistakes you make and can take into account special problems. To determine the best procedure for you to use, the therapist will consider the physical condition of the person you care for and the furniture and room arrangements in the home.

Transfers

Transferring a person in and out of bed is an important caregiver activity. It can be done fairly easily if these instructions are followed. Use the same procedure for all transfers so that a routine is set up. Any time the person with AD resists you, consider whether the person understands what you want him to do and whether he feels safe. Fear and confusion are often the cause of resistance. During transfers people may feel more vulnerable and may resist out of fear or not knowing where they are going. A skillful confident approach and a willingness to work with the person will go a long way toward cooperation.

Helping Someone Get Into Bed

To help the person in your care get into bed, use the following steps:

1. Have the person walk toward the bed and then turn around, as if he were going to sit in a chair. He should feel the mattress behind both legs.

2. Have the person slowly lower himself to a seated position on the bed, using his arms to control the lowering.

3. Have the person sit on the edge of the bed.

4. Lift legs into bed (one at a time may be easier).

5. Help him lie down with head on pillow.

6. Help him slide legs into center of bed (moving one leg at a time may be easier).

Turning in Bed

It is common for the frail elderly to have trouble turning over or getting in and out of bed. These tips may help:

- A satin sheet or piece of satin material tucked across the middle of the bed can make it easier for the person to turn over.

- Flannel sheets and heavy blankets can make it more difficult to turn over.

Helping Someone Get Out of Bed

To help the person in your care get up from bed, explain and repeat the following steps:

1. Have the person bend knees up. Place feet flat on bed.

2. Have the person turn onto his side. Reach arm across his body to assist rolling.

3. Help him move his feet off edge of bed.

4. Tell him to use his arms to push himself into sitting position. (A bedside rail fastened to the side of the bed may help.)

Helping a Person Stand

Help only as much as needed but guard the person from falling.

1. Have her sit on the edge of the chair or bed. Let her rest a moment if she feels lightheaded.

2. Instruct the person to push off with the hands from the bed or chair armrests.

3. Position your knee between the person's knees.

4. Put your arms around the person's waist or use a transfer belt.

5. Keep your back in a neutral position.

6. At the count of "1-2-3," instruct the person to stand up while pulling the person toward you and pushing your knees into the person's knee if needed.

7. Once she is upright, have her keep the knee locked straight.

8. Support and balance her as needed.

NOTE If during a transfer you start to "lose" the person, do not try to hold the person up. Instead, lower the person to the floor.

NOTE A transfer belt is a belt placed around the waist of a disabled person that is used to secure the person while walking.

Transferring from a Wheelchair to a Car

Be sure the car is parked on a level surface without cracks or potholes.

1 • Open the passenger door as far as possible.

• Move the left side of the wheelchair as close to the car seat as possible.

• **Lock the chair's wheels**.

• Move both footrests out of the way.

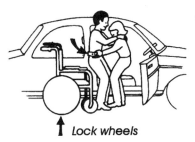

↑ Lock wheels

◀*2* • Position yourself facing the person.

• Tell the person what you are going to do.

• Bending your knees and hips, lower yourself to his level.

• By grasping the transfer belt around his waist help him stand while straightening your hips and knees.

• If his legs are weak, brace his knees with your knees.

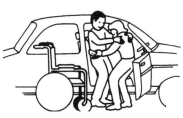

◀*3* • While he is standing, turn him so he can be eased down to sit on the car seat. GUIDE HIS HEAD so it is not bumped.

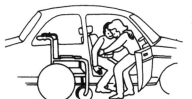

◀*4* • Lift his legs into the car by putting your hands under his knees.

• Move him to face the front.

• Put on his seat belt.

• Close door carefully.

Falls and Alzheimer's Disease

NOTE "In 2003, almost 13,000 people 65 and older died from a fall. Of those who survive a fall, 20-30 percent will suffer debilitating injuries that affect them the rest of their lives" (Source: National Safety Council, Report on Injuries in America, 2003). This is why it is essential to try to prevent falls from occurring.

There are many reasons why older adults are at risk of falling, including the effects of medications, slowed reaction times, brittle bones, stiffness, and lack of flexibility and impaired vision. Due to changes in the brain that are caused by Alzheimer's disease, people with AD are at especially high risk of falling. Slower reaction time, difficulty recognizing changes in the height or depth of a step, for example, can lead to tripping and falling. Changes in balance and coordination combined with poor memory can make it difficult for a person with AD to both get from one place to another and avoid hazardous objects at the same time. He may miss a step while looking for a door or trying to listen to someone's conversation. You can reduce the risk of falling by modifying the environment, as outlined in *Preparing the Home*, p. 25. You can also try to help the person in your care remain as active and flexible as possible. It is also important to provide appropriate footwear and review medications with his doctor. But if in spite of your efforts the person does fall, the following guidelines will help you to respond.

Fear of Falling

A person with AD, even in the early stages, probably will have subtle changes in walking ability that will become more severe as time goes on. This can create difficulty with balance. If the person has other illnesses, the problems may be more severe. It is natural that he will fear falling.

To help the person in your care feel more confident, adaptive devices such as walkers or canes can be useful, but you will have to remind him to use these devices. Bring the cane or walker to the person when he has forgotten it. Exercises that you can do with the person in your care may improve his balance. Remember, before starting any type of exercise routine, get advice from your physician. Start slowly with only moderate effort. Give the care receiver time to build strength and stamina. Any amount of exercise helps reduce risk, and the benefits of exercise are cumulative, so find a way to make it easy and enjoyable to exercise. Exercise is a particularly effective way to reduce depression.

And finally, everything said here about the benefits of exercise also apply to the caregiver. *You* need exercise as much as the person in your care. Find a way to make it part of most days.

If the Person in Your Care Falls

When you suspect a broken bone, follow these steps:

- If the person cannot move or use the injured limb, keep it from moving. Do not straighten a deformed arm or leg.

- Support the injured part above and below the site of the injury by using folded towels, blankets, pillows, or magazines if the person cooperates.

- If the person is face down, and breathing is adequate, leave the person in the same position.

- Keep the person warm with a blanket and make the person as comfortable as possible.

- Call 911.

If you suspect the person in your care has fainted:

1. Do not try to place the person in a sitting position. Instead, immediately lay him down flat.

2. Cover him with a blanket if the room or floor is cold.

3. Do not give fluids.

4. Call 911 if person is having difficulty breathing, not breathing, or not responding to your voice and touch.

> **NOTE** If *you* fall, you may not be able to rely on a person with AD to help you or to call for help. You may want to consider enrolling yourself in a First Alert type service, that you can activate in such an emergency.

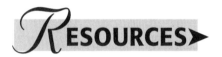

RESOURCES

American Academy of Orthopaedic Surgeons
6300 N. River Road
Rosemont, IL 60018
(800) 346-AAOS (800-346-2267)
www.aaos.org
Offers a free booklet Lift It Safe *on lifting procedures for home-based caregivers.*

If you don't have access to the Internet, ask your local library to help you locate a Web site.

Special Occasions and Challenges

Special Occasions and Challenges

An important part of caring for a person with Alzheimer's disease is to help her to continue to engage in activities that have special personal or family meaning (this is not a big problem in the early stages.) With suitable support, she will be able to enjoy taking trips, participating in events that mark significant moments in family and community life, and going to events such as college reunions and revisiting places that are part of her own personal history quite far into the disease.

Special Situations

Joyous celebrations such as weddings, baptisms, and birthdays and distressing events such as funerals may all occur during the years the person is ill. Some of these events will be expected and you will have time to give thoughtful consideration to the decision about if and how to include the person with dementia. Other events will occur suddenly and you will need to decide quickly how to respond.

There is no "right answer" to the question about whether to include or exclude the person with dementia. Experts, friends, and family may not all agree on the best plan, but there are some questions you can ask yourself to help you decide. How will the abilities the person has lost and those that are retained affect his participation? Will it be meaningful to the person to be present at a given event? Will it be meaningful to others that the person with dementia is present regardless of his ability to understand what is happening?

Issues to Consider

The Stage of Dementia

In general a person in the early stage of Alzheimer's can handle interacting in a social situation. However, he will need support to be able to take part in and enjoy events outside his regular daily routine. The person in the early stage may need to be reminded of the names and his relationship to the people he is talking to. If word-finding is a problem, a supportive person nearby may be able to fill in the gaps. A trip to the bathroom may require a guide.

A person in the middle stage will need continuous support to attend an event that is not in a setting designed to meet his needs and to keep him safe. There is the danger that the person will be overwhelmed by the unfamiliar activity, misunderstand what is happening, or wander away. If incontinence is already a symptom it should be dealt with in such a way that it does not embarrass the person with dementia or interfere with the comfort of others.

In the late stage it is unlikely that a person with dementia will be attending events outside his place of residence.

Will the Person Enjoy Being Present?

If you think that the person will be able to enjoy being present because there is food and music, even if he does not understand exactly what is happening and does not recognize the other guests, the experience may be enjoyable. On the other hand, if the environment will be overwhelming or overstimulating, the person may become agitated.

- Will there be a place where the person can rest or take a break from the activity?

- Will the behavior of the person with dementia interfere with the experience of others?

Arrangements necessary to provide for the person's safety and comfort:

- If the event is not near the person's home, will the trip be too tiring and confusing?

- Do you need to bring an aide or other support person along? How expensive will the additional services be?

- Will it be necessary to stay at a hotel or the home of a friend or family member?

- Will adaptive devices such as a raised toilet seat or commode be available?

- Will the person with dementia wander around or wake up in the middle of the night and disturb others?

- Will the person with dementia feel uncomfortable in an unfamiliar setting?

- If the event is near the person's home, and getting the person to the event and back home again is not too difficult, you may feel more willing to "risk" bringing him.

- If the person cannot walk, is the bathroom wheelchair accessible?

- Is there a ramp or an elevator for people who cannot climb steps?

 Tip Bring along a change of clothes, items to distract the person if he gets restless, and something you are sure he will enjoy eating.

Will You Enjoy Having the Person Present?

Will you be so distracted by the arrangements for the person with dementia that you will not be able to enjoy the event yourself? It is entirely reasonable to consider your own needs, the meaning of the event to you, and how the presence of the person with dementia will affect you. Will it be worth all the effort to include the person in the particular activity?

As with all activities you plan for a person with dementia, don't try to do it on your own. Get help for all aspects of the arrangements and expect the unexpected.

And don't be disappointed if the person does not remember the event or having taken part in it. The good feelings created by being there may persist beyond the memory of the actual event. On the other hand, if things did not go well, they may soon be forgotten.

Can You Be Flexible?

Can you be flexible and change the arrangements at the last minute? Even the best of plans may need to be changed, or canceled entirely, if symptoms of the illness interfere. The person with dementia may become too agitated, behave inappropriately, or be unable to get ready in time to go, perhaps making you or someone else miss the event as well. If it turns out that it is not feasible to include the person with dementia, can you accept this as a result of the symptoms of the illness?

> **NOTE** People with dementia can be unpredictable. They do not do this on purpose. A plan that seems to make perfect sense may turn out poorly. And that doesn't mean that you made a mistake.

Joyous Occasions

There is probably a wider range of behavior that is acceptable when the mood of the occasion is joyful. People will probably be tolerant. A person with dementia who says or does the wrong thing will not disturb the atmosphere and may even add to the general festivities. Even if Grandma comments in a loud voice, "I don't know where they got this food," her remark can be taken with humor and understanding.

 Note: Always remember that the person with dementia is doing the best he can and don't criticize or shame him for his efforts.

Family Events

There are many family events that the person with dementia can participate in and enjoy. Experiences that are not "once in a lifetime" occasions but still require extra planning so the person with dementia can participate occur fairly often.

Activities that had meaning to the person before he became ill, such as playing baseball with the family, may still be enjoyable if you plan the event to take into account his remaining strengths and his limitations. For example, he may not be able to keep score or follow all the rules, but may be glad to throw the ball.

Some events may be especially enjoyable. Everyone in the family may welcome having Grandma along on a visit to the local zoo or museum or to see her grandchild in a kindergarten play. Grandpa can still go to the ballgame if you remember to take his special needs into account. Perhaps he should only go for a few innings. Be prepared to leave early even if it is hard for you to miss the rest of the game. Remember that extra time should be allowed to get there, so there is no stressful last-minute rush.

Some settings are easier to take than others. Perhaps the person you are caring for will not be able to sit quietly through an entire movie or a concert, but you don't need to rule out everything that is a little out of the ordinary.

Driving

Can the Person with Dementia Continue to Drive?

Driving is a major issue for people with dementia and their relatives. In all but the most urbanized areas, a car represents independence and may even be a necessity. But it is also a threat to the lives of the driver, the passengers, and those he may inadvertently hit if he is no longer a safe driver.

The question about the ability of the person with dementia to continue to drive comes up as soon as the diagnosis is made, and sometimes even before. Others may have noticed changes in the way the person handles the car, if he is able to follow directions, and how often he gets lost on the way to familiar places. Sometimes friends and relatives will refuse to ride in the car if the person with dementia is driving, and give a variety of excuses rather than say that they no longer feel safe with her behind the wheel.

There are many reasons that family members are reluctant to acknowledge that the person with dementia should no longer drive. Perhaps no one else is able to drive and no other means of transportation is readily available. They may want to protect the feelings and dignity of the person with the diagnosis of dementia. They may explain minor accidents by blaming the situation or other drivers.

Stopping driving need not be a sudden event. It is best if it is a step-wise process. In the early stages of dementia, the person may be safe driving in very familiar areas. Perhaps someone can drive behind him once a month to check his driving, and let you know if he feels it is still safe. In cases of disagreement, an on-road driving test may help the family, and possibly the person with dementia, accept that she is no longer competent to drive.

While the reluctance to take the keys away is understandable, not taking them may lead to serious injury to the person with dementia or to other people. Laws differ from state to state regarding the responsibility of doctors and family members to have the driving skills of a person with dementia evaluated and then, if necessary, to have the license revoked. All states allow health professionals and others to report individuals they believe to be medically unfit to drive due to dementia or other conditions. This reporting is anonymous. After a report has been filed the subject of the report will be notified. She then must prove she can still drive safely. She may have to retake the standard on-road driving safety test.

Signs that the person is no longer a safe driver include:
· braking often for no apparent reason
· missing signs and signals
· getting angry easily
· swerving in and out of lanes and getting lost in familiar places
· crashes
· dents on car
· not reacting to traffic signs
· driving too fast or too slow
· poor judgment
· turning around to talk to the person in the back seat and forgetting that he is driving

How to Stop the Person from Driving

If the person with Alzheimer's is unwilling to stop driving when it is apparent to others that it is necessary, then someone needs to step in and make the decision for him. It is generally more emotionally difficult for men to stop driving than for women. You can't talk the person out of his reactions, which are totally understandable from his perspective, even though they may be painful for you to tolerate. You need to listen with empathy and an open heart to the effect of this loss on this person.

You may feel guilty for having to take the steps necessary to assure that the person with dementia stops driving, but it may be a matter of life and death and the decision should not be avoided.

It may be easier for a respected professional, such as the doctor, or family friend to inform the person of the end of his driving career. This may feel more comfortable to the family who will be the receivers of the feelings of anger, loss, and even betrayal from the person with dementia. But if necessary you may have to hide the keys, disable or even sell the car to prevent the person from driving.

Some caregivers continue to let a person with dementia drive because they have never learned how and don't want to feel trapped at home. If there are no good alternatives you may have to learn to drive, which may feel frightening to you, especially if you have been reluctant to do so for many years. On the other hand, it may be empowering to acquire a new skill. It will be safer than relying on the person with dementia to drive you. You may not have been considering relocation, but if there are no reliable and convenient means of transportation available to you, you may need to take this step.

NOTE Many states ensure transportation to necessary medical care for Medicaid recipients. Check with your local Medicaid office to see if the person in your care qualifies.

Transportation

There is a network of transportation services, public and private, that will pick up the disabled and the elderly at their homes. These services rely on vans and paid drivers and run on a schedule to specific locations. Free transportation is available from community volunteer organizations, although most public services charge on a sliding scale (see *Resources,* p. 246).

Community transportation services are provided by:

- religious organizations
- civic clubs
- the local American Red Cross
- the Area Agency on Aging
- local public transportation companies

Travel

Caregivers often have trouble deciding whether it is possible or worthwhile to travel with the person who has AD. It will require a lot of advance planning and knowledge of local resources. The person may function at a much lower level in unfamiliar surroundings than at home. Time changes, language, and strange people may cause distress. You will be required to provide a great deal more support while traveling than you do at home. Caregivers are often disappointed that the person with AD does not remember the trip on which they expended time, energy, and financial resources. However, some trips are essential, and others may give you pleasure. You may choose to spend the extra energy to include the person in your care on the trip, and it is possible that both of you may enjoy many aspects of the experience. Some group tours and cruise lines cater to the elderly or disabled traveler.

TRAVEL PLANNING

If you, as the primary caregiver, are traveling for an extended period, consider investing in a long-distance pager with a toll-free pager number so you can be reached in case of emergency.

Travel Emergencies

In the event of an emergency abroad, contact American Citizen Services (ACS) in the foreign offices of American consulates and embassies.

American Citizens Services will assist with:

- lists of doctors, dentists, hospitals, and clinics
- informing the family if an American becomes ill or injured while traveling
- helping arrange transportation to the United States on a commercial flight (must be paid by the traveler)
- explaining various options and costs for return of remains or burial
- helping locate you, the caregiver, if you are traveling when a family member becomes ill

Travel and Living Wills

If a person becomes disabled with a life-threatening illness while traveling, the medical personnel in foreign countries may not accept the validity of an advance directive (or any other form a personal attorney has drawn up). If a person is traveling and has an illness that requires breathing devices or other life-prolonging treatments, it may be impossible to end the treatment without a medical evacuation back to the United States. However, there a few basic precautions you can take to ensure that a person's wishes are carried out:

- Take a copy of the living will on the trip. Let any other traveling companions know where it is packed.
- Take health-care directive documents with you.
- If traveling in the United States, consider signing the form used in the state where you might be traveling.

TRAVELING ABROAD

When traveling in tropical countries, use the standard traveler's rule: boil it, peel it, cook it, or forget it!

Traveling with Medications

Traveling with medications should not stop you and your care receiver from enjoying travel in the United States and abroad. Some tours or cruise lines require a note from the doctor stating that the person is fit to travel. Here are some tips when traveling with medications:

- Bring enough medication to last through your trip plus some extras.

- Pack your meds in a carry-on bag—luggage can stray or become lost.

- Keep all medication in original containers with original prescription labels.

- Make a list of the medications the person takes, and why, with brand and generic names. Make a copy and pack one copy separately.

- Make arrangements for refrigerating the medication.

- If intravenous medication is used, carry a used-needle container.

- Bring the person's insurance ID card, plus instructions for accessing a physician where you are going.

- Bring the doctor's name and contact information, in case of emergency.

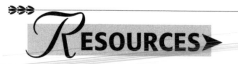

Driving

AAA Foundation for Traffic Safety Senior Driver
http://www.seniordrivers.org

AARP Driver Safety Web site
http://www.aarp.org/families/driver_safety

The Hartford
http://www.thehartford.com/alzheimers

National Highway Traffic Safety Administration
Telephone: 1-800-327-4236
http://www.nhtsa.dot.gov

Transportation and Travel Resources

Centers for Disease Control and Prevention
(877) FYI-TRIP (394-8747)
Fax requests: (888) 232-3299
www.cdc.gov
Provides recommendations on vaccinations and health data for travel to specific countries; also provides information about diseases such as malaria and yellow fever.

Consular Information Program
Bureau of Consular Affairs
State Department
(202) 647-3000 for automatic fax
(202) 647-5225 for recorded messages
www.travel.state.gov
Provides travel advisory information and emergency assistance. Ask for a complete set of Department of State, Bureau of Consular Affairs publications including "Medical Information for Americans Traveling Abroad."

Easter Seals
230 West Monroe St.
Chicago, IL 60606
(312) 726-4258 (tty) (800) 221-6287
www.easterseals.com
Provides a Transporation Solution for Caregivers booklet and accompanying video with tips and safe, creative solutions devised by both family caregivers and professionals, which are designed to ease transportation challenges.

If you don't have home access to the Internet, ask your local library to help you locate any Web site.

Part Three: Additional Resources

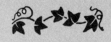

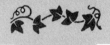

Caregiver Organizations

Alzheimer's Organizations*

There are Alzheimer's associations throughout the United States and many other countries that provide a variety of valuable services to people with AD and their family members. We suggest you contact an association in your community to begin learning about the resources available.

The Alzheimer's Association
(800) 272-3900 (312) 335-8700 www.alz.org
The Alzheimer's Association is the leading voluntary health organization in Alzheimer care, support, and research. It provides helpful information and links to local chapters. If you need to talk, their toll-free, 24-hour, seven-days-a-week help line (800-272-3900) provides reliable information, referrals and support in 140 languages. The local chapter in your community provides core services to families and professionals, including information and referral, support groups, care consultation, education and safety services.

The Alzheimer's Disease Education and Referral Center (ADEAR)
(800) 438-4380
www.alzheimers.org
Center Web site will help you find current, comprehensive Alzheimer's disease (AD) information and resources from the National Institute on Aging (NIA). Provides information in English and Spanish.

*Because of limited space we cannot list all organizations. Exclusion does not mean they are not valuable.

Alzheimer's Foundation of America
866.AFA.8484 (toll-free) 866.232.8484 (toll-free)
www.alzfdn.org
Toll-free hotline provides information, counseling by licensed social workers and referrals to community resources across the nation. The hotline operates during regular business hours-Monday through Friday, 9 am to 5 pm (EST). At all other times, please leave a message and your call will be returned.

Alzheimer's Research Forum
www.alzforum.org
Provides information for families and professionals with links to organizations worldwide.

Fisher Center for Alzheimer's Research Foundation
(800)-ALZINFO.
www.alzinfo.org
One Intrepid Square
West 46th Street & 12th Avenue
New York, NY 10036
This organization provides a comprehensive list of professionals and services in your area. They have information and resources that will help you make the right choices in insurance and financial planning, legal matters, and medical and end-of-life care.

Mayo Clinic Alzheimer's Disease Center
www.mayoclinic.com
The Mayo Clinic Alzheimer's Disease Center has easy to understand, practical in-depth information on Alzheimer's and caregiving.

Medline Plus
www.nlm.nih.gov/medlineplus/alzheimersdisease.html
A service of the US National Library of Medicine that posts the latest research findings.

International Alzheimer's Organizations

Alzheimer's Association of Australia
P. O. Box 4019
Hawker ACT 2614 +61 (2) 6254 4233
Dementia Hotline 1800 100 500
www.alzheiners.org.au
Alzheimer's Australia is the main organization providing support and advocacy for the 500,000 Australians living with dementia.

Alzheimer's Disease International
64 Great Suffolk St.
London SE 1 OBL UK +44 20 79810880 (Fax) +44 20 79282357
www.alz.co.uk
The umbrella organization of Alzheimer associations around the world. The site has links to member countries.

Alzheimer Europe
www.alzheimer-europe.org
An organization that aims to improve the care and treatment of Alzheimer patients through intensified collaboration between its member associations. Provides information in many European languages.

Alzheimer Society of Canada
(800) 616-8816 (toll-free within Canada) (416) 488-8722
www.alzheimer.ca
The Alzheimer Society is the leading not-for-profit health organization working nationwide to improve the quality of life for Canadians affected by Alzheimer's disease and advance the search for the cause and cure. Located in every province across Canada and in over 140 local communities. Provides information in French and English.

International Caregiver Information and Support Organizations

AUSTRALIA

Carers Australia

www.carersaustralia.com.au

(800) 242-636

Carers Australia represents the needs and interests of caregivers at the national level by

- *Advocating for carers' needs and interests in the public arena.*

- *Influencing government and stakeholder policies and programs at the national level through conducting research and pilot projects, giving presentations, and participating in a wide range of inquiries, reviews, and policy forums.*

- *Networking and forming strategic partnerships with other organizations to achieve positive outcomes for carers.*

- *Providing carers with information and education resources, undertaking community activities to raise awareness, and coordinating and facilitating joint work between the state and territory organizations on matters of national significance.*

CANADA

Canadian Caregiver Coalition

www.ccc-ccan.ca

The Canadian Caregivers Coalition helps identify and respond to the needs of caregivers in Canada. Links to organizations helpful to caregivers.

Caregiver Network, Inc.
(416) 323-1090
www.caregiver.on.ca
Based in Toronto, Canada, CNI's goal is to be a national single-information source to make your life as a caregiver easier.

UNITED KINGDOM

Carers UK
www.carersuk.org
The leading campaigning, policy, and information organization for carers; membership organization, led and set up by carers in 1965 to have a voice and to win the recognition and support that carers deserve.

UNITED STATES

Family Caregiver Alliance
690 Market Street, Suite 600
San Francisco, CA 94104
(800) 445-8106; 415-434-3388 Fax: (415) 434-3508
www.caregiver.org
E-mail: info@caregiver.org
Resource center for caregivers of people with chronic disabling conditions. The Web site provides information on services and programs in education, research, and advocacy.

National Alliance for Caregiving
4720 Montgomery Lane, 5th Floor
Bethesda, MD 20184
www.caregiving.org
The Alliance is a non-profit coalition of national organizations focusing on issues of family caregiving.

National Family Caregivers Association
10400 Connecticut Avenue, Suite 500
Kensington, MD 20895-3944
(800) 896-3650; (301) 942-6430
www.thefamilycaregiver.org
Email: info@thefamilycaregiver.org
The Association supports, empowers, educates, and speaks up for more than 50 million Americans who care for a chronically ill, aged, or disabled person.

Glossary

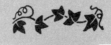

ஃ A

Acetylcholine: a neurotransmitter needed for memory and learning

Activities of daily living (ADL): personal hygiene, bathing, dressing, grooming, toileting, feeding, and moving from bed to chair or to bath, etc.

Acute: state of illness that comes on suddenly and may be of short duration

Adult day care: some centers have a dementia-specific program in a supervised environment where seniors can be with others; social models do not have medical supervision, which is provided by the medical model so it can meet the needs of a more frail and impaired population

Advance directive: a legal document that states a person's health care preferences in writing while that person is competent and able to make such decisions; the Living Will tells what treatment to provide while a Health Care Proxy allows someone to make decisions for the ill person based on the wishes of the ill person. Issues concerning life support should be decided as early as possible so all caregivers know the person's wishes

Age-associated memory impairment: normal forgetfulness that increases with age

Amnesia: complete or partial loss of memory

Amyloid plaques: a characteristic finding in the brains of Alzheimer's disease patients consisting of clusters of beta-amyloid protein

Analgesics: medications used to relieve pain

Anticholinesterase: a class of drugs frequently prescribed to patients with Alzheimer's disease, which have some modest positive effects for some patients

Anti-inflammatory drugs: a class of drugs including aspirin, ibuprofen

Anxiety: a state of discomfort, dread, and foreboding with physical symptoms such as rapid breathing and heart rate, tension, jitteriness, and muscle aches

Apathy: a condition in which the person shows little or no emotion or initiative

Aphasia: a speech problem that sometimes occurs in patients with Alzheimer's disease or other cognitive illnesses

Apolipoprotein E (apoE): a protein whose main function is to transport cholesterol; the gene for apoE is on chromosome 19; there are three forms of apoE: E2, E3, E4. E4 is associated with about 60% of late-onset Alzheimer's disease and is considered a risk factor for Alzheimer's disease

Artificial life-support systems: the use of respirators, tube feeding, intravenous (IV) feeding, and other means to replace natural and vital functions, such as breathing, eating, and drinking

Assessment: a determination of physical and/or mental status by a health professional based on established medical guidelines

Assisted living: a residential care setting that combines housing, support service, and health care for people typically in the early or middle stages of Alzheimer's disease; was initially mainly for active seniors who need some assistance

Assistive devices: any tools that are designed, fabricated, and/or adapted to assist a person in performing a particular task, e.g., cane, walker, shower chair

Atrophy: the wasting away of muscles or brain tissue

Autopsy: examination of a body organ and tissue after death. Autopsy is often performed (upon request) in order to confirm the diagnosis of Alzheimer's disease

B

Behavioral symptoms: in Alzheimer's disease, these are the symptoms that relate to action or emotion, such as wandering, depression, anxiety, hostility, and sleep disturbances

beta-amyloid: a sticky, starch-like protein that is the main component of amyloid plaques

Blood pressure: the pressure of the blood on the walls of the blood vessels and arteries

Body language: gestures that serve as a form of communication

Body mechanics: proper use and positioning of the body to do work and avoid strain and injury

C

Calorie: the measure of the energy the body gets from various foods

Caregiver: the person or persons who provide assistance to a patient in performing the ADLs, IADLs, and other support as needed; often an Alzheimer's disease patient's primary caregiver is the patient's spouse, sibling, or child

Cataract: a condition (often found in the elderly) in which the lens of the eye becomes opaque

Catheter: a rubber tube for collecting urine from a person who may be bed-bound and/or has become incontinent; there are a number of different kinds that are suitable for various needs

Central nervous system (CNS): the CNS includes the brain and the spinal cord and is the control network for the entire body

Cholinesterase inhibitors: medication that slows the breakdown of acetylcholine that is used to treat AD

Chronic: refers to a state or condition that lasts 6 months or longer

Cognition: brain functions involving thinking, remembering, learning, reasoning, and planning

Cognitive rehabilitation: techniques used to improve the functioning of individuals whose cognition is impaired because of physical trauma or disease

Computed tomography (CT) scan (pronounced "cat scan"): a type of X-ray that can give a health care professional two- and three-dimensional views of an internal organ or bodily tissues; in Alzheimer's disease patients, CT scans of the brain are sometimes used to support the diagnosis

Congregate living: a type of independent living in which elderly people can live in their own apartments but have meals, laundry, transportation, and housekeeping services available

Conservator: a person given the power to take over and protect the interests of one who is incompetent

Contracture: shortening or tightening of the tissue around a joint so that the person loses the ability to move easily

Decubitus ulcer: pressure sore; bedsore

Dehydration: loss of normal body fluid, sometimes caused by vomiting and severe diarrhea

Delusions: firmly held false beliefs that cannot be changed by explanation or evidence that they are not true

Dementia: a progressive decline in mental functions

Dementia with Lewy bodies: type of dementia that involves confusion, falls, and hallucinations as well as signs of Parkinsonism

Depression: a psychiatric condition that causes feelings of sadness and emptiness and hopelessness

Disorientation: a cognitive disability in which the senses of time, direction, and recognition become inaccurate and difficult to distinguish

Diuretics: drugs that help the body get rid of fluids

Durable Power of Attorney: a legal document that authorizes another to act as one's agent in legal and financial matters and is "durable" because it remains in effect even when the person becomes disabled or mentally incompetent

Durable Power of Attorney for Health Care Decisions: a legal document that lets a person name someone else to make *health care decisions* after the person has become disabled or mentally incompetent and is unable to make those decisions

Dysphagia: difficulty with or abnormal swallowing

⌇ **E**

Edema: an abnormal swelling in legs, ankles, hands, or abdomen that occurs because the body is retaining fluids

Estate planning: a process of planning for the present and future use of a person's assets

⌇ **F**

Frontotemperal dementia: dementia associated with difficulty making plans and setting goals, language trouble, personality change, and an unawareness of any loss of mental ability

৯ G

Gait: a person's manner of walking; people in the later stages of Alzheimer's often have "reduced gait," meaning they may lose the ability to lift their feet as they walk; changes in gait may also occur early in the illness but are very subtle

Gene: the basic unit of heredity; a section of DNA coding for a particular trait

Geriatric: refers to people 65 or older

Guardian: the one who is designated to have protective care of another person or of that person's property

৯ H

Hallucination: false perceptions of things that are not really there

Hippocampus: a small, "S"-shaped structure in the brain that appears to play a major role in the process of making memories

Hospice: a program that offers a range of services to people nearing the end of life and to their families that allows a dying person to remain at home while receiving professionally supervised comfort and care as well as emotional support

৯ I

Incontinence: involuntary discharge of urine or feces

Instrumental activities of daily living (IADLs): activities such as using the telephone, paying bills, cooking, and shopping; differs from basic activities of daily living

Intravenous (IV): the delivery of fluids, medications, or nutrients into a vein

Involved: a term used to describe the side of the body most affected by a disease, operation, or medical condition

৯ L

Long-term memory: that phase of the memory process considered the permanent storehouse of infomation

৯ M

Magnetic resonance imaging (MRI): A painless procedure that takes a picture of a person's brain, which can help in the diagnosis of Alzheimer's disease

Medic-Alert®: bracelet identification system linked to a 24-hour service that alerts the caregiver in the case of an emergency

Medicaid: a public health program that uses state and federal funds to pay certain medical and hospital expenses of those having low income or no income, with benefits that vary from state to state

Medicare: the federal health insurance program for people 65 or older and for certain people under 65 who are disabled

Mild cognitive impairment (MCI): forgetfulness that is worse than normal for one's age but that doesn't include problems common in dementia like confusion; the severity of MCI falls between that of age-associated memory impairment and early dementia

Mini-Mental State Examination: a test of mental status used to check for any basic cognitive impairment

N

Neuron: the basic cell of the nervous system responsible for controlling the actions of the body by signaling to other neurons

Neurofibrillary tangles: abnormal structures formed inside nerve cells in AD; their presence causes dysfunction of nerve cells and eventually kills them; neurofibrillary tangles are composed of tau protein

Neurotransmitter: a chemical that sends messages between nerve cells

Nursing home: a licensed facility that provides room and board and a planned, continuous medical treatment program, including 24-hour-per-day skilled nursing care, personal care, and custodial care

Nutrition: a process of giving the body the key nutrients it needs for proper body function

O

Occupational therapy: therapy that focuses on helping people to perform the activities of daily living such as personal hygiene, bathing, dressing, grooming, toileting, and feeding

Ombudsman: a person who helps residents of a retirement or health care facility with such problems as quality of care, food, finances, medical care, residents rights, and other concerns; these services are confidential and free; this person is called the "patient advocate" in the hospital

Oral hygiene: the process of keeping the mouth clean

ॐ P

Paranoia: a mental disorder characterized by false beliefs that others intend to do harm or are not trustworthy

Passive suicide: killing oneself through indirect action or inaction, such as no longer taking life-prolonging medications

Pathogen: a disease-causing microorganism

Personal care: assistance provided by another person to help with walking, bathing, eating, and other routine daily tasks

Physical therapy: the process of relearning walking, balancing, and transfers or to support healing after an accident or injury

Plaques: local buildup of amyloid-B in the brain of AD patients, damaging nerve cells and destroying connections between them

Posey: a vest-like restraint used to keep a person from getting out of bed

Possible AD: a diagnosis of Alzheimer's disease giving a moderate suspicion that the person has Alzheimer's disease

Pressure sore: a breakdown of the skin caused by prolonged pressure in one spot; a bed sore; decubitus ulcer

Probable AD: a diagnosis of Alzheimer's disease giving a high suspicion that the person has Alzheimer's disease

Prognosis: a forecast of what is likely to happen when an individual contracts a particular disease or condition

Protein: the product of gene expression; proteins are the molecules that do much of the work in the body such as creating structures, using and storing energy, and transmitting signals

Psychometric tests: tests to measure cognitive function

ॐ R

Range of motion (ROM): the extent of possible passive (movement by another person) movement in a joint

Rehabilitation: after a disabling injury or disease, restoration of a person's maximum physical, mental, vocational, social, and spiritual potential

Respite care: short-term care that allows a primary caregiver time off from his or her responsibilities

ॐ S

Sedatives: medications used to calm a person

Shock: a state of collapse resulting from reduced blood volume and/or blood pressure caused by burns, severe injury, pain, or an emotional blow

Speech therapy: the treatment of disorders of communication, including expressive language, writing, and reading and communication required for activities of daily living

Stroke: sudden loss of function of a part of the brain due to interference in its blood supply, usually by hemorrhage or blood clotting

Sundowning: unsettled behavior of a person with AD evident in the late afternoon or early evening

Support groups: groups of people who get together to share common experiences and help one another cope

Symptom: sign of a disease or disorder that helps in diagnosis

T

Tau protein: abnormal protein that in AD piles up inside nerve cells, forming neurofibrillary tangles that directly lead to death of nerve cells

Tranquilizers: a class of drugs used to calm a person and control certain emotional disturbances

Transfer: movements from one position to another, for example, from bed to chair, wheelchair to car, etc.

Transfer belt: a device placed around the waist of a disabled person and used to secure the person while walking; gait belt

Transfer board (Sliding Board): polished wooden or plastic board used to slide a person when moving from one place to another, for example, bed to wheelchair or commode

Trapeze: a metal bar suspended over a bed to help a person raise up or move

V

Vascular dementia: dementia from blood vessel disease usually caused by a series of tiny strokes

Vital signs: life signs such as blood pressure, breathing, and pulse

Void: to urinate; pass water

Index